DR FRANCES GOODHART
AND LUCY ATKINS

HOW
TO
FEEL
BETTER

D0064248

piatkus

To our parents: Celia and William Goodhart,
and Sue and Peter Atkins

PIATKUS

First published in Great Britain in 2013 by Piatkus
This paperback edition published in 2015 by Piatkus

1 3 5 7 9 10 8 6 4 2

A CIP catalogue record for this book
is available from the British Library.

To protect the anonymity of the people quoted in this book,
their names and personal details have been changed.

The recommendations given in this book are solely intended as education
and information. Check with your doctor before changing or stopping
any treatments or medications.

ISBN 978-0-7499-5820-6

Typeset in Aldus and The Sans by M Rules
Printed and bound in Great Britain by
Clays Ltd, St Ives plc

Papers used by Piatkus are from well-managed forests
and other responsible sources.

MIX
Paper from
responsible sources
FSC® C104740

Piatkus
An imprint of
Little, Brown Book Group
Carmelite House
50 Victoria Embankment
London EC4Y 0DZ

An Hachette UK Company
www.hachette.co.uk

www.piatkus.co.uk

Praise for *How to Feel Better*

'Every patient – and every patient's supporters, be they relative, partner or friend – will find help from this book. From the start of a phase of medical intervention, right through to the struggle to get out of it and back on with life, Frances and Lucy have broken the entire process into understandable sections, and demystified the process. By giving a structure to feelings that you might otherwise only be dimly aware of, or not at all until too late, it informs and guides the reader through the complex geography of appointments, illness, treatment and recovery. As a succinct guide to the journey through illness, it has the makings of a classic. I warmly commend Frances and Lucy on a sympathetic and above all practical guide'

Professor Justin P Cobb,
Chair, Section of Orthopaedics,
Imperial College London

'This book is a great companion for people living with long-term conditions and their families. It gives simple, practical advice for those faced with the challenges of illness, such as dispelling their worries and giving coping strategies for managing stress. I like the examples from people who have experienced illness and these will be inspirational to others. I would recommend this book to anybody with a long-term condition and their families, as it shows it is possible to put quality back into life after a diagnosis'

**Dr Barbara Conway, British Heart Foundation
Cardiovascular Specialist Nurse,
Doctor of Nursing, County Durham &
Darlington NHS Foundation Trust**

'For doctor and patient alike, those familiar with serious illness recognise that the associated mental struggle, stress and uncertainty are at least as great a challenge as the physical illness and its aftermath.

How to Feel Better is a detailed, practical guide that understands these problems and provides practical evidence-based solutions. The insight and experience of Dr Goodhart are easily apparent through the many thoughtful tips and strategies, whilst the key themes and ideas are related by the authors in a style that is accessible, without being patronising. The authors draw on many patient vignettes that resonate with my own clinical practice. Indeed, the handbook is as helpful to the thoughtful doctor as to his or her patient. This is an important, well-balanced and serious contribution that will provide the interested patient, carer and professional with new perspectives, tips and insights'

Robin P Choudhury DM FRCP
Professor of Cardiovascular Medicine,
University of Oxford & Consultant Cardiologist,
Oxford Heart Centre

'It is extraordinary that no one has written a book like this until now. It is designed to help you take off where the medical profession left off. Inventive, practical and authoritative, this book will help with the obvious and unexpected challenges of recovery after illness'

Dr Suzy Cleator BM BCh MRCP FRCR PhD
Consultant Clinical Oncologist and Honorary Senior Lecturer,
St Mary's and Charing Cross Hospitals,
Imperial Healthcare NHS Trust, London

'This is a really timely book. It puts together much if what I have gleaned over the years and try to tell my patients in a rush in 8 minutes! The advice is sensible and manageable, and phrased in a way that doesn't make you want to give up before you have started. A great resource to dip in and out of as you come across different hurdles in convalescence'

Rosie Haining, Edinburgh GP

'This book is a joy – thoughtful and funny, practical and realistic. It takes the whole potentially terrifying process of medical investigation and treatment and breaks it down into manageable pieces, with well-researched tactics and tips to help at every stage. Designed to help both patients and carers, it avoids jargon and highlights the all-important psychological issues which are so often underestimated. Having a long-term illness brings many challenges, emotionally as well as physically. With this book comes the promise of feeling just a little less overwhelmed'

Dr Sarah Jarvis, GP and medical broadcaster

Dr Frances Goodhart is a consultant clinical psychologist with twenty years' experience of working with individuals and families who are coping with life-threatening illnesses. She worked for several years as an NHS Macmillan Consultant Clinical Psychologist in Oncology and Palliative Care. Dr Goodhart's patients include men and women of all ages, and she supports not just the patient, but their families and carers too. She also provides psychological consultation and supervision to medical and nursing colleagues. Dr Goodhart's work has been published in academic journals and presented at national and international conferences. She has a BA (hons) in Experimental Psychology from the University of Oxford, an MSc in Clinical Psychology from the Institute of Psychiatry, London University, and a doctorate in Clinical Psychology (D. ClinPsych) from City University. Dr Goodhart lives in London with her husband and three children.

Lucy Atkins is a well-known health journalist. For the past fifteen years she has written health features for the *Guardian*, the *Weekend Telegraph* and the *Sunday Times*, the *Sunday Express*, *The Times*, *Red*, *Woman and Home*, *Grazia* and the major mother and baby magazines. She is also the author of *Blooming Birth* (Collins, 2005) and *First-Time Parent* (Collins, 2006 and 2009). Lucy has been a media commentator on health and family issues, online, in podcasts, and on radio and on television. She currently lives in Oxford with her husband and three children.

ACKNOWLEDGEMENTS

Enormous thanks to: Anne Lawrance and the fabulous team at Piatkus; The British Heart Foundation – in particular, Kevin Fitzpatrick, Darlington Coronary Heart Club, Gordon Wilcock, Dr Barbara Conway, Adrian Hurley, Dr Melissa Sanchez; The Stroke Association – in particular, John Hillman, Ealing Stroke Club, Pat Badger, Tewin Over 50s Social Club; Professor Nadina Lincoln, Dr Anna Sorensen, Dr Catherine Hood, Dr Michelle Kohn and Kelly McCabe at the London Oncology Centre's *Living Well* programme. Huge thanks also to Bungie Snow, Trilogy Boot Camp, Zina Sabovich, The Wellcome Trust, Jothy Rosenberg and Francis King. Above all we are grateful to the many other people who so generously gave up their time to tell us about their experience of illness, injury and recovery, whether in person, by email, phone or even Twitter. Finally, thank you – as always – to our families: Jim, Josie, Beatrice and Kitty, and John, Izzie, Sam and Ted.

CONTENTS

INTRODUCTION

'The end of an illness is not always in sight when the doctor's visits cease. Very often the weeks of convalescence which follow the turning point of a malady are almost as trying to the patient and his family as the illness itself, and they are certainly, although in a different way, quite as critical.'

British Medical Journal, 1911

A serious health problem is like an earthquake with you at its epicenter – it's frightening and noisy, it rocks your foundations and shakes you up, familiar structures collapse around you. You make it out of the wreckage – health professionals bring you to safety and patch you up . . . but then they leave. You're supposed to be 'feeling better', you're meant to be 'getting your life back', but your landscape has changed – the landmarks and structures look different, possibly even unrecognisable. You know you're supposed to rebuild it all, but you're still shaken up. Even when the physical symptoms are under control, it can take a while to really *feel* better. You need help, but your rescue team has gone. You feel very alone. What now?

Well, that's where this book comes in. If you have had a heart attack, a stroke, cancer, surgery of any kind, or been hospitalised for a serious illness such as pneumonia, or something out of the blue, like a car accident, then this book is for you. It is for anyone whose health has unexpectedly taken a blow. It provides the tools and strategies to help you rebuild yourself.

In days gone by, there was a whole phase between illness and recovery, called convalescence. For at least three centuries this was taken very seriously indeed. Scientific papers – sometimes entire books – were written about it. There were convalescent spas and rest cures, 'wellness' regimes, bath chairs, water cures, tonics, sanatoria in the Swiss Alps. Doctors, nurses and carers debated the tiniest details of convalescent care, right down to how to lay the dinner tray. Nobody was expected to just 'bounce back'.

In today's quick-fix, high-tech world, the notion that feeling better takes time has somehow been lost. Nowadays, we are meant to 'Get Well Soon', pick up where we left off, move on, get our lives back, be our 'old selves' . . . The Victorians and Edwardians may have enjoyed hanging around in bath chairs, but we have jobs to hold down, mortgages to pay, households to run – and no domestic staff. We also have the benefits of modern medicine: effective pharmaceuticals, state-of-the-art scans and blood tests, follow-up consultations, physiotherapists. When our bodies are fixed – or at least stabilised – we are expected to feel 'better'.

If only it were this simple. The truth is that when your body takes a serious knock, so does your mind. Even if you look fine you may feel, deep down, as if your foundations are cracked. You may feel worried, confused, lonely, depressed, unsupported or overwhelmed. You may be grappling with ongoing physical challenges such as disability, pain, the side effects of treatment, sleep problems, fatigue or muscle weakness. You may have practical concerns about finances, work or plans. Or you may simply be trying to 'adjust'. If any of this sounds familiar, then you are far from alone. Countless people struggle, often in silence, long after the physical symptoms of their illness or injury have been controlled.

In 1927 an American doctor called John Bryant wrote in his

book, *Convalescence*, that 'most of our large hospitals display in their corridors direction signs, some of which bear the legend THIS WAY OUT. But these signs too seldom tell the patient whither the hospital portals lead.' This sense of disorientation is just as strong today as it was in 1927: those hospital 'portals' still lead us into the unknown. We may be given information leaflets, follow-up appointments and rehab instructions, but we don't get bespoke, in-depth, ongoing care or a crash course in rebuilding our lives.

That is why we wrote this book. It is about understanding what happened to you when the 'earthquake' hit. It is about learning simple, practical ways to cope with the tricky emotions that surface. It is not about turning back the clock, creating a society of invalids or re-opening the sanatoria. Nor is it about navel-gazing and feeling sorry for one's self. It is simply about finding a path through what Dr Bryant called 'the space between illness and health'. It is about understanding what has happened, and learning ways to cope. This is the 'modern art of convalescence' – for convalescence is just as vital today as it ever has been.

All the strategies in this book are evidence-based (that is, they are backed up by rigorous scientific studies). They don't always make their way into rehabilitation courses or leaflets but they are essential if you want to survey the damage, sift the 'rubble' and rebuild yourself – from the inside out. Your life may never be exactly the way it was, but take the strategies in this book seriously and you won't just 'cope', you'll thrive.

A word for carers

You may have been catapulted into a role that you never imagined, and certainly didn't ask for. You may not feel entirely confident about this. In fact, the whole 'carer' thing may seem completely daunting right now. Your life has changed too – and this can throw up a lot of different emotions. The truth is that it's perfectly normal for you to go through many of the emotions that your loved one is experiencing: to feel stressed, anxious, depressed or simply exhausted.

If you can read the whole of this book, please do. The techniques here can really help you to cope too. Otherwise, look at the 'Notes for Carers' sections at the end of each chapter. It might also help if you tell yourself – right now – that you don't need to be the perfect carer, just a 'good enough' one. Caring for someone is a learning process. You are bound to have ups and downs. You're likely to make mistakes. And there will almost certainly be days when you think, 'I just can't do this any more.' You, too, need practical ways to cope with tricky emotions – whether they are yours or those of the person you are caring for. This book, in short, is for you too. For once, your needs are not being overlooked.

ONE

DOCTOR'S ORDERS

HOW TO GET THE BEST FROM YOUR MEDICAL TEAM

> *'Sir John Broadbent entered my room and again I felt the relief of a strong efficient man devoting his whole mind to my care ... He focussed his whole attention and his entire self upon my needs. I felt his learning and his experience, and I saw that he paid attention to the smallest detail – even the position of my pillows. On one occasion he seized me tightly in his arms and seemed to literally hold me together when I appeared to be falling to pieces.'*
>
> **Sir Francis Youngblood,** *Treatise Within:*
> ***Thoughts During Convalescence***, **1913**

Doctors may have loomed large in your life recently. How you interact with them, and cope with their suggested treatments, can make a huge difference to how you feel.

Many of the most basic barriers to feeling better come down to the practicalities of dealing with health professionals, new regimes or medical setbacks. There are numerous challenges, but if you learn how to manage them calmly and with a clear head, and communicate well with your medical team, life can improve dramatically.

What is 'feeling better'?

You might think the answer to this question is pretty blooming obvious. But good health is actually a complicated concept. Health is not, in fact, something you 'get' or 'lose'. There may have been times in your life when you felt you 'had' your health, but the truth was that things went wrong then too – even if it was only the odd bout of flu or a sprained ankle. It is therefore worth thinking just for a moment about what 'feeling better' means for you. This will give you a clear sense of what you can expect of yourself – or where you (realistically) hope to get to.

It might mean:

- Feeling that you are back where you were before this health crisis.

Or

- Feeling that you have enough independence so that life seems doable again.

Or

- Feeling that you can cope with ongoing health issues and/or ongoing contact with a medical team.

Or, indeed, anything else. It just has to be meaningful to you.

Leaving hospital

Most people can't wait to get through the hospital exit. They see it as an end point – they'll be 'better' or 'cured' or 'safe' when discharged.

Although going home is certainly a milestone, it is rarely the end of the story. What catches many people by surprise is that going home can actually be quite frightening and disorienting.

Suddenly, you are away from this powerful medical support. You are alone, perhaps with only a distant follow-up appointment on the horizon. Without the whole reassuring structure of hospital life, you might feel as if you are gazing out at the wreckage of your life. You don't want to turn back but the task of rebuilding your familiar structures seems truly daunting, if not impossible.

❝I found it hard leaving intensive care, with one-to-one nursing, and being moved on to a general ward, but that was nothing compared to being sent home. I'd become used to the hospital observations – temperature, blood pressure, fluid intake, "How are you today Catherine?" Not having those formal measurements to prove that I was OK, and not having someone to answer my questions and put my mind at rest, was frightening. It took me weeks, really, to feel confident again.❞

Catherine, 29, had a car accident

It doesn't help that you may be dealing with some complicated new challenges at home: medications, exercises, dietary regimes, lifestyle changes, repeat prescriptions to keep track of, benefit forms to fill in.

Of course, you may be lucky enough to get great follow-up care.

❝I could contact my specialist heart nurse with any question or concern, I had regular check-ups at the hospital, my doctor was informed about every hospital visit, and I can't fault the cardiac rehabilitation course I went on – it was brilliant.❞

Tom, 70, had a heart attack

Equally, however, you may find yourself adrift on the margins of a system that doesn't seem to know who you are.

❝I never saw the same doctor twice at my outpatient follow-up appointments. I had to repeat everything and I never felt any of the doctors I saw then were really very interested in me. It felt like they had pulled the short straw having to do the outpatient clinic and they just wanted to get it over with as soon as possible. I had to talk about my difficulties with bowel continence each time I went to a follow-up but I got very little advice or support. Eventually I insisted that I see the consultant who knows me and my case, at which point I felt that the situation started to improve.

Oliver, 57, had bowel cancer

The good news is that there are many effective ways to communicate your needs and find support. You don't have to feel abandoned, scared and alone when you leave hospital – that's just unreasonable after what you've been through.

TIP

'Best before ...'

If you are given a time frame for your recovery – when you can expect to walk again, or drive, or return to work – try to remember that this is a rough guide only. You, personally, could take more (or less) time to achieve this goal. Doctors often give out time frames because patients want them, but they are only estimates based on averages. The danger is that if you don't recover in a given time frame you end up feeling 'worse' than other people – weaker, less competent, less healthy. You start to think that you'll 'never' get better.

It is therefore a good idea to treat recovery a bit like the 'best before' date on a food packet: the food won't instantly shift from palatable to poisonous the minute the clock passes midnight on the date that's stamped on the package. It's just a guideline. Similarly, you are not a failure if you haven't hit your recovery target on an exact day. Equally, resist the temptation to view your doctor's 'get better by' date as a challenge (competitive people are likely to find this particularly hard). Try not to think, 'Right, I'm going to better/halve that date.' You probably won't. The danger is you'll push yourself too far too fast, overdoing it, and setting yourself right back.

How to manage follow-up appointments

There are all sorts of highs and lows involved in follow-up appointments. You can even out the journey a lot by learning a few simple survival tactics.

Before you go

Unless you have anxiety-management superpowers, a medical follow-up is likely to involve at least some degree of worry. Appointments can:

Dredge up bad memories of traumatic or difficult events. You might have to go back to the very hospital where you were treated, or see staff who treated you at the time. You will have to think about your health in detail since your last appointment, and this can be difficult if you feel you haven't made 'enough' progress. Or you may have to think back to how you were when things were very bad, in order to make comparisons with how you feel now.

⟨To get to the outpatient clinic from the hospital entrance I have to walk along the corridor that I was wheeled through after my stroke. Even though I have been well for years, entering that corridor still makes my heart beat faster and my breath tighten in my chest.⟩

Hitesh, 69, had a stroke

Highlight current symptoms It is surprisingly easy for this to turn obsessive. As you 'tune in' to your body, you start to notice things you'd normally ignore (for example, your heart beating fast, or tiny temperature changes, or aches, pains, niggles and twinges). You start to worry that something's wrong. Then you start to dread the appointment. What will the doctor tell you? What does your future hold? Psychologists actually have a term for this: 'hypervigilance'. It's surprisingly common even in the calmest, most rational person.

Nerves, symptom-watching and worrying can stop you from getting the most out of your appointment, whether talking or listening. It is therefore a good idea to get on top of this rather than just thinking, 'it's part of the deal'.

Try this: manage your follow-up nerves

When the appointment letter lands on your doormat and you feel a stab of worry, ask yourself the following questions:

- 'What exactly is worrying me?' Is it just the clinic appointment letter that has made you anxious or do you have physical concerns or symptoms?
- 'What's the evidence?' If you do have physical concerns, what specific symptoms do you have that suggest there is a problem? (It's good to think this through, then you can take this detailed information to your appointment.)
- 'How did I cope last time I had an appointment?' Think back – were there things you did last time that you shouldn't do this time? (For example, Googling your symptoms? Asking an unreliable friend to give you a lift and being late?) Was there anything that helped you to cope? (Taking a loved one with you for support? Meeting someone afterwards for coffee?) Can you do this again?

Once you've worked out what, exactly, is worrying you, you can use strategies to minimise the unpleasant effects of nerves.

Your nerve-management toolbox

There are long-, medium- and short-term nerve-management tools. You'll probably need all three.

In the weeks or days before the appointment

Prepare for tension If you are aware of how anxiety affects you (see Chapter 2, page 38), then you can prepare yourself, and others, for the fact that it's likely to happen. You can explain, clearly, to loved ones (or even colleagues) how anxiety makes you behave so that they have the 'heads up'. This can help you to bypass a lot of conflict and confusion that will only make you more wound-up. You could also suggest ways people can help (for example, maybe they could avoid telling you to 'stop worrying', or asking you why you're so quiet).

Manage your worry symptoms Relaxation strategies such as visualisation or mindfulness techniques are useful (see page 94) at the end of the day when the worries kick in. You can also use 'quick fix' strategies for when you suddenly think about the appointment, and your heart races (see page 48). You could start a worry diary (Chapter 2, page 41) in the run-up to the appointment. This will help with future appointments – you'll recognise your worries and be able to anticipate them.

Exercise 'It is possible ... that you can do without a doctor entirely; that is without a human doctor for I wish you to put yourself under the kindly care of Dr. Sunshine, Dr. Fresh Air, Dr. Exercise, and Dr. Regularity,' advised the Victorian magazine columnist 'Medicus' ('The Mind and The Health', *Girls Own Paper*, 1881–2). Clearly, you aren't going to eschew the doctor in favour of wearing flannel, drinking Vichy water, and dusting flowers of sulphur inside your stockings, as one Victorian doctor advised, but building some fresh air, exercise and daylight into your life will help you to manage the physical tension that comes with appointment-related anxiety. See Chapter 10, Exercise and Well-being, for more ideas.

Make practical arrangements Planning makes you feel more in control. It will help you to concentrate on the appointment. Things to consider: who, if anyone, is going with you? Where do you have to go? (Do you know exactly where the outpatient clinic is and how you'll get there?) How long will the journey take? What will happen after the appointment? Plan a treat for afterwards, too, if you possibly can.

Watch out for Thought Traps Your thoughts can be your worst enemy. This is an idea you will encounter throughout this book. For a full explanation of Thought Traps and how to tackle them see page 54. If you can spot unhelpful thoughts, and manage them, you are likely to feel much more in control. Common appointment-related Thought Traps include:

- Catastrophising: 'I've made no progress. I'm worse than ever. There is no hope for me.'
- Fortune-telling: 'The doctor's going to say I have to come back into hospital/have more surgery/treatments.'
- Mind-reading: 'They won't want to hear about my ongoing pain – they're too busy for my silly problems.'

Build your 'case for the defence'

Example: 'The doctor's going to say I have to come back into hospital/have more surgery/treatments.'

What's the evidence? Has the doctor already told you this? Do you have a letter saying this? Has someone phoned to warn you in advance? Do you have lots of unmanageable symptoms or have you been functioning well out of hospital? Why would a routine follow-up appointment change this?

What are the 'mitigating circumstances'? You are thinking this – almost certainly – because you're tense and worried. Can you recall other times when you have been tense and worried and found yourself fortune-telling like you are now?

Is thinking like this fair or helpful? No. The doctor has not told you this. This is a very scary thought, but it may not be fair. It is understandable to worry like this but try to think about other options as well – maybe you will be sent home with a clean bill of health or a minor adjustment to your treatment regime. It is easy – but unhelpful – to get stuck with your 'worst-case scenario' thought, so try to remind yourself of other possible outcomes.

Managing your thoughts like this probably won't make your 'follow-up nerves' vanish, but it will keep them under control.

Short-term nerve management

The day before the appointment:

Conduct your own health audit Write a brief list of any episodes of ill health or odd physical sensations you've had since your last appointment, as well as any physical milestones or times when you felt really well. No one needs a blow-by-blow account of every sniffle, but a clear outline of significant health changes or symptoms, how long they lasted and how you managed them, can be incredibly helpful.

Include a list of your medications At the end of your health audit, jot down what you're taking – how much and when (include over-the-counter medicines and herbal or other remedies).

Write a list of questions Consider what *you* want to get from this appointment. Are there areas of your ongoing treatment that you're unsure about or don't understand? Are there things you don't feel are working or symptoms that haven't been tackled? Do you need extra help? A brief list of questions will help you to stay focused. Your medical team will thank you for this.

The day of the appointment

Turn up! This sounds ludicrous, but it's often tempting to just skip the whole thing. If you feel OK, you may tell yourself it's not necessary. If you feel ill, you may simply be too scared to show up. Drs Sunshine and Regularity are no substitute for the real thing. If the meeting at work seems too vital to miss, or you suddenly think you can't burden your neighbour with yet another lift to the hospital – stop! This is avoidance. When it comes to follow-ups, avoidance is playing with fire. For every follow-up appointment that feels like a bit of a waste of time, there will be another where an aspect of your treatment is significantly improved, or where you need an important medical intervention. Even if you are fine, it can be helpful for your medical team to know what you're like when you are well (for example, what your normal blood pressure or heart rate is, what your normal blood count or weight is).

Take your lists – take your health audit, and your questions.

EXPECT DELAYS

It's called a waiting room for a reason. You know delays are likely. But try to act on it this time. Give yourself time, don't schedule the appointment between two important meetings. Remind yourself what really matters here: your health – rather than letting the fury about the organisation of the clinic, or your missed meetings, build up like a pressure cooker.

❝The first couple of times I went to my outpatient appointment at 1.30 pm I had not made any arrangements for someone else to pick up my sons from school at 3.30. I ended up making frantic phone calls just as I was being called into the consulting room – not the best start. Now, when I have a clinic appointment, I arrange for them to go on play dates with friends who know I may be late. This way I don't get so wound up if clinic runs late.❞

Carla, 33, had a spinal injury

TIP

Take distractions with you

When you take a toddler to the doctor's surgery, you take books, toys, or anything that will stop a nuclear meltdown. This approach is helpful for adults too. Assume there will be no entertainment in the waiting room. Take a newspaper, book, crossword or sudoku, a letter to write, your iPod, a smartphone containing the emails that need responses. Be busy.

Try this: focus

If your entertainment runs out, or you can't concentrate, or you forgot to take anything, try this calming and distracting mindfulness technique:

1 Focus on the details of the room Look at the patterns in the flooring, notice the shape of the chairs, the changing shade of colour on the wall, the exact shape of the lights. Look at everything as if you're an alien, seeing it for the first time. Or as if you're going to be tested on it afterwards: be rigorous and curious.

2 Focus on what you can hear – not the details of the conversation next to you (unless gripping), but on the different levels of noise: the loudness of the voices near you, the background hum of the traffic, the patter of raindrops against the window, even the whisper of your own breathing. It can help to close your eyes while you do this.

3 Focus on your body – in particular your breathing. Shut your eyes and focus on the flow of air into your nose and out through your mouth. Notice what happens to your body as you breathe in – your chest, tummy and shoulders rising, how the air flowing from your nose into your lungs feels, and so on. Do the same for the out-breath – notice how your shoulders and tummy drop back down again, how your muscles unwind, how your lungs deflate.

4 Thoughts will pop into your head – they may be worrying thoughts about symptoms, or how you'll cope in the appointment, or organisational thoughts about everything else you should be doing, or just random thoughts. Treat them all the same way: acknowledge the thought ('there's a thought about the shopping/an organising thought'). Don't try to push it away or squash it, but also don't let it lead you down a spiral of other thoughts. Without judging yourself ('Why can't I just focus on my breathing? I'm useless at this!'), try to refocus – on the room, the sounds, your breathing. You'll have to do this repeatedly – but keep doing it.

The appointment itself

As you walk into the doctor's room, you may suddenly feel small. It can seem as if that doctor, right now, holds the key to all your hopes and fears. Many people have harsh or unrealistic expectations of themselves when they go in: 'I mustn't cry', 'I'm going to understand every word that's said to me', 'I'll challenge the doctor if I don't like what she says' or 'I have to put all the worry behind me.'

The truth is, you are unlikely to be at your most suave, eloquent or sharp-minded in your appointment. You may well get emotional. You may not understand what's being said to you. You may struggle to make decisions or remember things. Doctors are used to this; however, there are ways to get around this so that your appointment is as productive and unstressful as possible.

Coping with white coat syndrome

You sit down to talk to the doctor and things you've been obsessing on for weeks suddenly vacate your mind, leaving a gaping hole. The hole fills up immediately you leave the doctor's office, but when you're in there you are pretty much blank. This is 'white coat syndrome'. White coat syndrome can also affect your blood pressure, pulse, breathing rate and produce other annoying symptoms. It's surprisingly common.

6I am a scientist, I am not stupid and I do try to prepare for medical follow-ups. But the moment I sit down in a chair opposite a doctor I seem to lose my intellect and become emotional. I think it is just the reminder of how much I owe them. The consultant is very good; he gives me time to compose myself and then the appointment continues.9

Simon, 54, had acute pancreatitis

Doctors are well aware of white coat syndrome, but they can't mind-read. So if yours kicks in you could:

Tell the doctor It can help to just say 'I'm really nervous' or even 'I'm suffering from white coat syndrome'. Sometimes just getting it off your chest can calm you down, and help you to remember what you wanted to say.

Take your list Have your list of questions you want to ask easily accessible – you don't want to be scrabbling around for a scrap of paper at the bottom of your bag.

Take a friend Having a second set of eyes and ears in the room can give you a different perspective later. It can also help you to retain information. If you've told the other person your concerns (or at least written them down), they can help you get them across if and when the blankness descends. They can also help, afterwards, when you're trying to remember what the doctor said, or when you're worrying about something that was mentioned.

6My husband came with me to my first appointment with the cardiology team. I am so glad he did, because as soon as the doctor mentioned surgery I panicked. I imagined myself on the operating table. He, in contrast, actually listened to what was being said. He realised that they were talking about a more minor procedure of ablation and helped me to get things straight in my head and weigh up the pros and cons of the procedure afterwards. Honestly, without him I think I would have been a nervous wreck. 9

Isla, 67, had heart surgery

Remember that this is your one time When you are anxious, your sense of timing can go a bit haywire, so although you might be thinking to yourself, 'I've been jabbering on for hours,' you may have only taken up a few minutes of the doctor's time. You've got your questions. You need answers. Don't be intimidated by some warped sense of time or a fear of being a 'nuisance'.

6 I hadn't even had a chance to get my backside onto the chair before my consultant was telling me I was ready to go back to work. It was only four weeks after my heart attack and I was so taken aback I didn't ask a single question, just said, "Righto," and left the room. Luckily, I stopped for a cup of tea and the cardiac nurse found me and answered the questions I had. 9

Howard, 52, had a heart attack

TIP

Be realistic

Obviously, although it doesn't help to be intimidated by time, this is not a cosy fireside chat – it's a time-limited medical appointment. If you have a list of questions the length of your arm you are not going to get through them all. In advance, decide which questions are most important (pick the ones that will make the most difference in the weeks ahead). Write those at the top of your list. Also, think about who you are seeing and target your questions to their expertise; for example, you might want to discuss medication, treatment and what to expect with your doctor, but you could discuss rebuilding fitness, diet, mobility aids, returning to work or claiming benefits with team members, such as nurses, physiotherapists or occupational therapists. You may need to arrange separate appointments to do this.

Two more ways to make the most of your appointment:

1 Ask questions – even if they aren't on your list. Often one question will trigger others you didn't anticipate. If you don't understand something, then say so. It's perfectly fine to ask your doctor to repeat things or to clarify. Doctors these days go on communications courses, but still, there are going to be times when they inadvertently use jargon or get too technical.

2 Summarise. At the end, to check you understand, say something like, 'OK, so am I right in thinking the main points are ...' Or you could ask your doctor to summarise for you ('Would you mind summarising the main points so that I can be sure I've really understood?'). This sounds demanding, but it isn't really. The last thing your doctor wants is you going

away confused, or worse – not following important instructions or making bad decisions because you didn't get it. Your doctor wants you to understand.

Coping between appointments

Once the appointment is done, you may be left with all sorts of instructions or medications. Coping with this can be hard. Naturally, you are going to become more confident with new regimes as time passes. But you can speed this up so that daily health management stops feeling like such a burden. Again, it helps to have strategies up your sleeve.

Managing exercises

If you have been given physiotherapy, occupational therapy, speech therapy, psychological therapy, or a recovery manual to work your way through, then you are likely to have 'homework' (things you need to work on without the direct supervision of the therapist). You can:

Use a calendar Put it somewhere you'll see it – such as on the fridge door – and use it to keep track of your appointments or visits. You can also write your daily routine or treatments on it to remind yourself: go for a walk, take a rest (at a specified time).

Have 'homework' time Make it a set time every day and/or enlist someone to remind, support and motivate you. You could do your exercises each night while watching TV, or practise your relaxation techniques during a rest time, or exercise while walking the dog or as part of your commute. Building 'homework' into another routine activity really will help you to keep going.

Introduce variety Your therapist should be able to help with this. Doing something every day can become habitual but it can also become tedious, dull and, frankly, boring. You need to find ways to stay interested and motivated. If you have spent months walking round the same block or visualising the same desert island, try walking a different route – or even going swimming instead – and see if you can visualise a different place.

Keep a record If you note down each day what and how much you did, you'll not only have an accurate record to show to your therapist but you'll also be able to identify particular days or times of day when it is harder to fit your exercises in. You and your therapist will then be able to tweak things so that they actually work. It can also be very motivating to tick your own boxes each day.

Reward yourself Recovery can be painfully slow and some-times it's hard to see progress (you may also plateau, or have a setback – see page 27 for how to manage these). It is a good idea to reward yourself for the effort it's taking to stick with this therapeutic programme, whatever the results. See Chapter 4, page 121, about rewards and why they matter.

Managing medication

⁶My life seems to be ruled by medicines now. I have to take all sorts of different pills at different times, some with food, some without. It feels like my life has to be totally regimented and I am terrified of losing track.⁹

Fiona, 68, has arthritis, had deep vein thrombosis and now takes warfarin

Sometimes the logistics of taking all those pills can feel over-whelming. Here are some ways to make it run smoothly (and take up less of your time and mental energy):

Set timers Most mobile phones have an alarm function and many kitchens have an electric timer. You can set them to go off four hours later when your next dose of medication is due. You won't be living this regimented life forever – a new regime will become a familiar friend with time, but getting started takes planning and structure, plus the odd reminder.

Have one medicine cupboard Keep all your medication in it – prescription and over-the-counter. A kitchen cupboard (as long as it is secure) may be a better idea than one in the bathroom, especially if you have to take medicine with food several times a day. This way you won't have to hunt around for different medicines at different times or haul yourself upstairs before every meal.

Get a pill organiser Another obvious tip – but these magical plastic trays will really help you work out what to take and when, and they will monitor what you have taken. Once a week, you have to spend a boring few minutes doling out pills, but after that you avoid all the tedious bottle opening, and pill counting. Other gadgets may also seem silly but can be hugely helpful; for example, apparatus to push tablets out of fiddly blister packs, or to cut tablets in half. Small things can make a big difference to your levels of frustration.

Keep back-up medicine A couple of small pill organisers (see above) with a small amount of medication in your handbag or briefcase can stop you from missing a dose if you forget to take your medicine with you. You might keep a small amount in the office, gym locker or in your car, if those places are safe (that is, no one else can get at your medicines).

Try not to become obsessed Although it's important to follow pill-taking instructions, try not to feel completely ruled by them. Hospital-ward drug rounds don't always run on time. There are times when patients are given their medicines minutes, or even hours, late and occasionally medication slots are missed altogether. This is not ideal, but the point is that in the vast majority of cases a medication timetable is a guideline. If, from time to time, you take a dose late, or even miss a pill, it is not the end of the world. Similarly, medicine information leaflets can make scary reading, but you should take them with a heavy pinch of salt. Drug companies have to cover their backs. We all need to know what we are taking, but as you read the side effects, make sure to read the small print too: the statistics for any major side effect are usually minuscule. The drug would not be on the market if it damaged lots of people. However, if you do experience unexpected or unpleasant side effects from any of your medications, do talk to your doctor about them.

TIP

Find a helpful pharmacist

Pharmacists are often overlooked, but they can be one of your greatest assets. They are a marvellous source of information, wise advice and reassurance. They can give tremendous practical help (reordering repeat prescriptions, checking that all your prescriptions are compatible, arranging delivery of medication, recommending equipment to make life easier). Pharmacists can let you know when you need to reorder repeat prescriptions and can give you notice about when you need to go back to the doctor for another prescription. All this makes life so much easier. If you live in a place with more than one pharmacist, shop around to find one you like and trust, then make your pharmacist your best friend.

Coming off medication

Even if you do it slowly and carefully, coming off medication can be surprisingly unnerving. You might feel that by taking a tablet you're doing something active to improve your health. Stopping this can make you feel unexpectedly vulnerable. The first few days (sometimes longer) without your pill can trigger Thought Traps and a lot of worry. You might find yourself monitoring your body more closely than usual, worrying about physical sensations, such as your breathing or how hot you feel, or any physical twinges. Time and medical reassurance generally make you realise that it's OK, but this is rarely a speedy process. It helps to ask your doctor – and be very clear about – any possible symptoms or signs you should watch out for (see page 26). This way you can reassure yourself that you don't need to panic if you feel something. You may also need to watch out for unhelpful Thought Traps – it's easy to catastrophise, for example: 'I don't feel well, I really don't – this is because I've stopped the medication!'

> ❝Coming off my pills was surprisingly hard. It was the loss of a comfort blanket. I had to talk myself through it, I had to reassure myself that the reason I was stopping the pills was because the clot has gone. Each day I wake up I tell myself, "Yes, another day further away from the clot," and, as I work and exercise, I build up the evidence that the clot must have gone or I wouldn't manage what I do. It is as if each day I add another brick to my defence wall.❞
>
> **Ross, 54, had a pulmonary embolism**

Managing troubling symptoms

A troubling symptom is likely to trigger difficult thoughts, feelings and behaviours. While you are waiting for medical advice, it helps to have ways to stay calm.

Know what to look out for Talk to your medical team before you leave hospital or at an early follow-up so that you are clear about what symptoms you might experience and what to do about them. This won't cover all eventualities, of course, but having an idea about what they'd want to know can give you a framework. Try to get a sense of how urgent these symptoms might be (for example, 'we would want to see you within a couple of days if you noticed a loss of sensation' or 'chest pain lasting longer than 15 minutes and which does not respond to medication should be seen rapidly at A&E', or 'tell us if you have unexplained weight loss over a couple of weeks').

Ask your medical team if there is any way for you to get in touch for advice between appointments; for example, a quick phone call to a nurse specialist can put your mind at rest if you're not sure about something. Some staff may offer you their email address – this can be an ideal way to get the odd niggle off your mind without interrupting them too much.

Avoid Google Googling your symptoms is almost always a really bad idea. Google 'headache' and you've got a brain tumour, Google 'pain' and you're having a heart attack; however, visiting the recognised website of a well-established health charity, or calling their advice lines, or checking NHS Direct or NHS Choices online advice can be helpful.

Watch out for Thought Traps 'Catastrophising' is particularly common. If this happens, remind yourself: thoughts are *not* facts (see page 54). See if you can think about the other possible interpretations or explanations for your symptom.

Calm your body Remember, also, that worry has a direct effect on your body: your muscles tighten, your heart and breathing rates increase, your blood flow alters (see Fight–Flight, page 38). All of this can make a small symptom bigger. A walk in the park, a mindful meditation, slow breathing, a favourite magazine, book, TV show or computer game, a warm bath – or a combination of any of these can really help. You might find that the symptom you were worrying about goes away, or at least gets much less obvious – then you know it is at least in part to do with worry or tension.

❛ In the first few months after my heart attack I must have called the doctor ten times and gone to A&E three or four times. I didn't have the experience or knowledge to separate out the muscle twinge from a heart attack. Gradually, with experience, I realised that not all pain and twinges are dangerous. ❜

Eliza, 63, had a heart attack

Coping with setbacks

Feeling better is rarely a straightforward march towards magical wellness. Sadly, life doesn't parcel out its problems neatly – or fairly. You may have had more than your fair share of health challenges, but other problems may crop up too. When you face a setback, there are many things you can do to cope and keep going forwards:

Use your knowledge from last time If you have to go back to hospital, try to think about things – big and small – that you could do differently this time. If, for example, it took you a while to get things you needed last time (such as good books, or your music or reading glasses) make sure someone brings them for you as early as possible this time. If you had too many visitors last time, get a message out that you appreciate good wishes but cannot see too many people. If you felt that you did not get enough physiotherapy support last time, see if you could ask for more this time. If you were in pain when the nurses moved you last time, ask for a painkiller in advance this time. If you found it all confusing last time, could you ask the staff to explain things more clearly? Would writing things down help?

TIP

Use your experience

You have had to face and manage at least one health problem – possibly many more. This means that you actually have experience to draw on when handling this setback. You've probably had to face non-health-related problems in your life too – at work, with money or relationships. Many of the strategies you've used to overcome non-health-related problems also work during a health setback. You may be thinking 'I'm back at square one', but you are very far from that. Ask yourself:

- What did I do that helped me manage my recovery before that I could use again?

- What did I do that wasn't so helpful? (Are these things relevant now or would something else work better?)

- How do I cope generally when things go wrong in life – what worked? (Coping with a redundancy, financial problems, relationship difficulties, caring for a family member, bereavement, and so on.)

Find support It may be that you need to talk about how you are feeling; having a relapse or setback is hard to cope with. You may be able to get support from your family, friends or direct medical team, but there are also other specialist staff in hospitals to talk to. Ask the nurses on the ward if you can see a social worker, counsellor or psychologist. Most hospitals also have chaplains and other religious leaders to offer emotional and spiritual support. It's a good idea to take a (polite) 'nothing ventured nothing gained' attitude.

HOW AND WHEN TO TALK TO MEDICAL STAFF IN HOSPITAL

- Pick your moment. During the daily ward round or observation times, hospital staff are concentrating on you. This is a good time to talk to them. Be realistic about how much time you need. If your question really is brief just say, 'Can I please take a moment of your time?' But if your concerns are more complex, try asking if they could come back to talk to you when they have more time. Try to book yourself an appointment with them.

- Open with a (genuine) positive. If you're asking to change some aspect of your treatment, start with a comment on something that's working well, then move on to the thing you'd like changed or improved. Medical staff are only human, and if you recognise their efforts and strengths, they are more likely to be receptive to things that need changing.

- Enlist help. A friend or family member may be able to go and talk to the staff at the nursing station (always wait until they've finish their call or paperwork; just ask for a few moments of their time). If they don't know much about your situation, they may be able to point your friend/family member towards a staff member who does know you better.

- Represent yourself. If you are hospitalised for a long time (several weeks or more) there are often multi-disciplinary team meetings to consider your particular needs in more depth. You could ask to contribute to this yourself – either in person if you can, or in writing or by sending a family member or friend along to the meeting.

Dealing with Thought Traps

Your thoughts can be one of the hardest things of all to handle during a setback. Common setback Thought Traps include:

- Catastrophising: 'This is a disaster, I worked so hard to recover and it has all been for nothing. I coped before, but I will never manage this.'

- All-or-nothing thinking: 'If I am going to keep going in and out of hospital, my life might as well be over.'

- Filter glasses. These filter the bad news and explain away or ignore the good. 'The doctor says it was a minor stroke and I should make a good recovery. But I haven't noticed any improvement today and the doctor seemed very young, she was probably junior and doesn't really understand.'

- Fortune-telling: 'I will never recover from this.'

Build your 'case for the defence'

What is the evidence? You may have put your 'filter glasses' on. Are you only focusing on what has gone wrong? Are there, in reality, some things that have gone well or at least OK? Is the medical team talking to you about getting home even if they can't give you an exact date? Were you warned that setbacks might happen? Have you had a setback before? Are you jumping to conclusions or 'fortune-telling' without having all the information you need? Think of anything you could do to get more information.

Are there mitigating circumstances? You may be expecting yourself to manage this perfectly from the start, but actually this crisis is new to you right now. You may be physically weak, or in pain, or otherwise debilitated – those things are hard to handle. Facing a setback is frightening, demoralising and exhausting, so it is little wonder if you get caught up in some Thought Traps.

Is thinking like this fair or helpful? During a setback you are bound to experience uncomfortable thoughts and emotions – so try not to beat yourself up about this. But it's easy to get caught in Thought Traps that are harsh, unfair and unhelpful. Remind yourself that there are other ways of looking at this situation. Are you overlooking some other possible outcomes? Try to think about things you may have done well. Perhaps you can think of ways in which you've been strong, or ways in which you are coping, despite this setback.

* * * * *

Thankfully, we are a long way from the days when doctors would prescribe a move to a seaside sanatorium for rheumatism, dole out cough mixtures containing heroin, or strap on electroconvulsive devices to cure impotence. But at times it can feel as if you do have to make a massive leap of faith when it comes to trusting your medical team. It can feel as if you've handed over the reins and all you can do is blindly trust that the team know what they are talking about.

It is fair enough to feel nervous and to want reassurance and clarification. This is why communication – two-way communication – matters so much. If you can find ways to negotiate the health system, cope with nerves and uncertainties and setbacks, talk to medical professionals, and put their expert advice into practice without going mad, then you will be taking a massive step in the right direction. And that – of course – will make you feel a lot better!

NOTES FOR CARERS

'Give medicine and the food at the proper time by your watch, and note down any change you may observe whether for the better or the worse ... This ought to be shown to the doctor and may be of very great service to him.'

'On Nursing the Sick', Medicus, *Girls Own Paper*, 1880

When you are caring for someone, it is easy to feel sidelined. The focus, rightly, tends to be on the patient – but this can leave you, as the carer, feeling lost, uncertain and at times completely in the dark. When it comes to dealing with health professionals and hospitals, you need information, communication and clarity. Here are some ways to achieve this:

1 **Inform yourself** There is nothing more disempowering than being in the dark. As a carer you need information just as much as the patient does. If you can go along to (at least some) medical follow-up appointments or rehabilitation sessions, you may feel much more empowered. If you can't manage this, you could explore whether someone could take notes for you at these appointments; whether the medical team have any leaflets or handouts that would clarify what has been decided; or even whether you could speak to someone on the phone afterwards, to make sure you're fully informed of the medical side of things.

   Remember, you have a legitimate need for this information, so don't be afraid to ask questions. Ultimately, you all want the same thing. And if you are giving the best care you can at home, then you will make the medical team's job easier too.

2 **Try to find a medical 'ally'** It is common for carers to assume that the professionals are there only for the patient. But some of them are also there to support carers. See if you can

find someone in your loved one's medical team who is willing to give you information and support.

3 **Agree on your role** It is a good idea to have a direct discussion with your loved one about what help they actually need from you. Try not to make assumptions about what they want. If you have any choice, be realistic about what you can offer and try not to get pulled in to offering more than you can realistically do. Also, bear in mind that this situation is likely to change – this conversation shouldn't be a one-off.

4 **Share the load** You may feel as if you 'have' to do it all, but this can be the route to burn-out. Ask your loved one's medical team whether there are community health or social services professionals who can help or take on a particular aspect of the care. It's also worth thinking how to get the most out of the support you do find. When someone else is supporting your loved one, you could take the time to do something for yourself, rather than hanging around feeling you should be there 'in case they need anything'.

5 **Know you're not alone** There are 'carers' organisations both nationally and locally and great online support resources. (See Resources for the organisations you can contact.)

❝I don't think Joe would have opted for any aftercare following his heart attack. He wanted to forget about it and threw the leaflets away. But I got them out of the bin and said I was going to the cardiac rehabilitation group even if he wasn't. He did come with me in the end and it was really good for both of us. We learnt a lot and met people we are still friends with ten years on.❞

Libby, 61, wife of Joe, 62

COMFORT AND CONTENTMENT

HOW TO COPE WITH WORRIES

'Certain patients are made more comfortable and contented, worry less and take their food with keener enjoyment if they are given alcohol.'

'The value of alcohol as a therapeutic agent'
Proceedings of the Royal Society of Medicine, **1920**

Ah, those were the days. Modern therapeutic approaches to anxiety management tend not to involve booze, but the idea of comfort and contentment is still vital to feeling better. If you are worrying a lot, you will not be able to feel better and move on.

Few people get through a health crisis without some anxiety, and many feel anxious for a long while afterwards. Worry can be exhausting, debilitating and distracting. It can stop you from living the way you want to live. But there are really effective, simple ways to tackle worries so that you can move past them, and feel better.

Common post-illness worries

Worries kick in when we are dealing with uncertainty and change. Health problems bring plenty of both. If you are grappling with new treatments or regimes, health professionals or medical equipment, financial, emotional or physical changes, and changes at home, at work and in your social life, it is little wonder you're worried.

The most common health worries include:

- Worries about becoming ill again:

  ❝When I'm on my own I do get a bit panicky. I think, what will happen if I have another heart attack, will anyone find me, will I be OK?❞
  Antonio, 63, had a heart attack and surgery

- Worries about not coping or not getting better:

  ❝I worry about the fact that I still can't manage the stairs at home or have a bath. The physios tell me I will keep improving, but I end up wondering if this is it – if this is as far as I will get. I worry about what that will mean for my future and my independence.❞
  Jean, 75, had a stroke

- Worries about the loss of professional support:

  ❝I only see my physiotherapist once a fortnight. He's given me exercises to do at home but I worry that I am not doing them right. I also worry about new activities. I went on my dad's rowing machine last week but got myself wound up wondering if I was doing too much or the wrong sort of movement. I wish I could have a direct line to my physio 24/7.❞
  Olly, 29, broke his pelvis

- Worries about the impact on loved ones:

  ❝I worry about my husband and how this has affected him. He doesn't have the best of health himself, but since I've been ill he's had to do so much and I don't think he is really looking after himself properly. He says not to worry, but that just makes me worry more. 9

Virginia, 58, had a heart transplant

- Worries about roles and jobs, and things that need doing:

6 I run my own company, with eleven people working for me, and I worry about them and if I will be able to keep the company going. I know everyone personally. I know their families, I know their circumstances and I am terrified of letting them down. 9

Paul, 48, had a cycling head injury

- Worries about the future:

6 I know this is going to get worse and I am already quite disabled by it. I'm on my own and I can't see how I'm going to cope. 9

Susan, 61, has arthritis and a double knee replacement

- Worries about worry:

6 People tell me that I am very strong to have got through my treatment, but I am eaten up with fears. Then I get frightened that by worrying I will make my cancer come back. 9

Karen, 37, had skin cancer

THE WORRY VOLUME SWITCH

One clinical psychologist, Paul Gilbert, likens anxiety to a volume switch – often we just need to turn the worries down. He describes a herd of gazelles grazing happily – then a lion comes. The gazelles leap away as fast as their legs can carry them, jumping over obstacles, avoiding dangerous routes, putting as much distance as possible between themselves and those slavering lion jaws. When the lion has gone they simply get back to the business of grazing. There is no critical incident debrief or psychiatrist's couch. The threat is over. They're fine. Life goes on. The gazelles, in other words, can 'turn down the volume' of their fear almost instantly. Humans, less so.

You have faced a threat to your health (even your life). Some lucky people can indeed turn down the fear volume and move seamlessly on. But, sadly, most of us aren't quite so gazelle-like. The volume of the threat may have turned down since your health problem was at its peak, but the threat may still be perfectly audible. And you may still be responding to it. Perhaps it's your own voice critically saying that you should be doing something different. Or maybe it's coming from the outside: another TV report linking obesity to every known illness; a website that scares the living daylights out of you; a message from your body: tightness in your chest, a bloated tummy, a headache, a scary twinge.

The fight–flight response

❝I get caught in a spiral of worry about my health: I notice something physical – it can be really small like being slightly out of breath – and suddenly my body gets completely wound up. My stomach lurches, my muscles tense up, my mind starts racing and, before I know it, I have diagnosed myself with another heart attack.❞

Isobel, 59, had a heart attack

What Isobel is describing is the fight–flight response: a hard-wired reaction to fear that is an evolutionary thing. The threats that primitive humans faced were, on the whole, physical (a hungry lion, a marauding tribe). They required physical action – fight it, or run (the lion is coming! Spear it! No – run like a gazelle!). The physical symptoms of anxiety – butterflies in your stomach, fast breathing, racing heart, dry mouth, sweaty palms, flushed face, restlessness, the desire to get away/escape – are rooted in this threat response; however, modern-day threats – health problems, a relationship break-down, financial worries – are not generally solved by running away or fighting. Sadly, our bodies have not caught up with this reality. Our instinctive response to a threat is therefore still physical.

If you really did fight the lion with your bare hands or run away, then your adrenalin-primed body would use up that extra adrenalin for the fight or flight and settle back down quite quickly. However, when you respond to modern-day threats, you do not tend to 'burn off' the adrenalin.

Your fear volume is stuck on high because your body is still on high alert. This isn't harmful but it certainly feels unpleasant; it leaves you feeling edgy, tense, hot and sick.

THE FIGHT–FLIGHT BODY DECODED

When anxious (that is, threatened) your body releases a chemical called adrenalin – which primes you for 'action'.

- WHAT YOU FEEL: breathless, heart racing, jittery.
  WHAT'S HAPPENING: your heart rate and breathing rate are increasing to feed your muscles with a good supply of oxygenated blood – they're going to be working hard if you have to run or fight.

- WHAT YOU FEEL: nausea, butterflies in the stomach, lightheaded, dizzy.
  WHAT'S HAPPENING: your body diverts some blood flow from your digestive system and your brain towards your limbs, which need the blood more (because you don't need to think complicated thoughts or digest food – you need to RUN or FIGHT!).

- WHAT YOU FEEL: hot, sweaty.
  WHAT'S HAPPENING: if you're going to run or fight you might overheat, so your body is priming your skin to cool down.

- WHAT YOU FEEL: flushed – your face goes red.
  WHAT'S HAPPENING: your body sends the blood flow closer to your skin's surface to make use of this sweaty cooling system.

- WHAT YOU FEEL: blurred vision and headaches.
  WHAT'S HAPPENING: your pupils dilate to let more light in so that you can see the threat more clearly.

Finding ways to 'damp down' this fight–flight response stops the worries from taking over. These are useful skills for anyone at any stage of life, but when your health is under threat, and you are facing a lot of changes, they become pretty essential.

What are worries made of?

Like all emotions, worry can be boiled down to four elements:

- Worried thoughts:

> ❝I can hear myself wheezing when I take a breath in. I don't think I have fully recovered, I think there may still be fluid on my lungs. I think the hospital may have discharged me too soon.❞
>
> **May, 72, had a respiratory arrest after a chest infection**

- Worried emotions:

> ❝I feel anxious most of the time, a sort of low-level unease. But when I hear a siren it is as if I am transported back to the scene of my accident and I feel a petrifying, paralysing terror.❞
>
> **Kaya, 28, hit by a bus while cycling**

- Worried body:

> ❝I feel sick, hot and sweaty whenever I go to a follow-up appointment. I can be perfectly all right on the street outside, but the minute I walk through the entrance and see the pale green paint on the hospital walls my stomach flips and I find it hard to breathe.❞
>
> **Raymond, 50, had a kidney transplant**

- Worried behaviour:

> ❝I get so agitated at work, I never sit down for long, I'm always making the cups of tea in the office because I need to move around. Sitting still and concentrating are skills that I seem to have lost along with my hair.❞
>
> **Elizabeth, 38, had breast cancer**

You might notice that one or other of these worry elements is dominant for you. But your worried thoughts, emotions, body and behaviour are all bound up together, even if you don't realise it. If you can identify all four elements of your own worries, then you can find ways to turn down the volume.

Try this: keep a worry log book

Getting your worries down on paper makes them feel less stuck inside your head. This gives perspective – seeing worries in black and white can make them feel less personal.

How to do it: give yourself 15 minutes at the end of the day somewhere quiet where you won't be disturbed (but don't do it in bed, as it could disrupt your sleep. Do it before bedtime). Do this for one week. Make sure you can write things down.

1 Think back to an incident today that made you worry or feel anxious. Write down what the situation was and what was happening when you felt worried; for example, 'Listening to the radio, heard piece about possible closure of local A&E department.'

2 Now, write down what emotions you felt when the worry hit you; for example, 'worried, nervous, angry'. Use the worry scale 1–10 (see page 47) to help you to rate what level of worry you felt.

3 Note how it made you feel in your body: 'tummy tightened, dry mouth, clenched fists'.

4 Try to record the thoughts you had at that moment (the words that went through your mind at that time). If you can't remember them, imagine what your thoughts might have been; for example, 'That A&E probably saved my life – it can't be closed. The next nearest A&E is 10 miles away. What would happen to me if I needed to go there again?'

(Make a mental note to yourself to try to notice what you are thinking next time you feel nervous, worried or scared.)

5 Finally, write down your behaviour: what you actually did when you felt nervous; for example, 'shouted at the radio then turned it off, went into garden'.

You might pick up patterns ('my anxiety peaks when I have a follow-up hospital appointment', 'I get much more worried towards the end of the day when I am tired'). You might be able to spot changes ('my fear of meeting other people has gone from 8 to 6' or 'I used to fill a page a day with my worries but nowadays it might be a page a week'). This is a useful way to see how your worries work.

TIP

If you're 'worry free' one day ...

If there's a day where you can't think of a single thing that worried you, don't let this stop you from writing something down in your worry log book. Instead, do the same thing, but for a happy, positive, calm, exciting or peaceful situation. Write down the situation ('with friend, walking in the park'), thoughts ('she's enjoying talking to me about her situation, we enjoy each other's company. I can still be useful'), emotions ('happiness, pleasure, contentment'), physical sensations (some tiredness and achy muscles but generally relaxed, enjoying feeling of sun on skin'), behaviour ('strolling, smiling, chatting').

By doing this, you are training yourself to tune into the four elements; they are there whatever situation you're in, whether it's a happy one or an anxious one. Being able to tune in is the first step to noticing these elements when you worry (without your log book) and ultimately gaining some control over them.

The fear of facing the fear

Thinking about recording your worries may be making you feel even *more* worried. If, as you read this, you've been getting a bit hot, tense or edgy, thinking, 'I don't like the sound of this' or 'What good will this do?', you're probably someone who tends to distract yourself from uncomfortable or tricky thoughts and situations. You might believe that if you spend time sitting around thinking about worrying situations you'll just wind yourself up more – thinking about something worrying might even make it more likely to happen.

If you recognise yourself here, you're far from alone. This is a very common reaction to scary thoughts. And, you're right, in some ways: endlessly going over possible awful scenarios can trap you in a vicious circle of worry and fear. But simply trying to distract yourself from all anxiety – keeping yourself so busy that you block out all worrying thoughts – tends to leave you wound up, frenzied and ultimately exhausted. Distraction, in short, can be useful in some short-term scenarios (for example, in the doctor's waiting room) but it does not work in the long term. The trick is to find a middle ground – a balance between containing thoughts and tackling them head on. But that's easier said than done, of course.

'Don't worry about it'

Being told not to worry doesn't work – even if you've been given solid medical information that's supposed to be reassuring. The problem is that although plenty of people say 'don't worry about it' nobody really explains how to do this. How, exactly, do you keep those pesky, alarming thoughts from leaping out and kicking you in the gut?

❝ The doctors say I am healthy and I mustn't worry. But I do worry. I worry about it several times a day, seemingly for no reason at all – I can be watching TV or in the supermarket and a little worry about my artery pops into my mind. And every time I get a headache I panic. I picture my blood clot dislodged from the artery and going up into my brain. If only I could have proof that the clot had disappeared completely I would be a new woman. 🍷

Amaya, 47, had a TIA (mini stroke)

Try this: bunny rabbits

1 Do not think about bunny rabbits. Stop it, don't think about them, don't picture them, don't let them into your mind – not even for a second.

2 What did you think about? Instantly? Yes – floppy ears, fluffy little tails, bouncing and hopping . . .

Keeping so busy that you do not let yourself worry is impressive, and it can squash some minor worries for good. But when it comes to major worries, this strategy is less successful. Usually, the minute you let your guard down the worry springs back up at you. Even if you only let yourself think about it for a split second it's enough to trigger that primitive fear reaction.

🍷I don't let myself worry. Every time I start to worry I get up and do some exercise. I try to tire myself out so I don't have the energy to worry. It does work, I exhaust myself – till bedtime that is – when my head hits the pillow – it's like, zing! I'm wide awake and worrying again. 🍷

Gary, 54, had a heart attack

The other end of the scale: obsessing

Your brand of worry may, of course, lurk at the other end of the scale. You obsess about things that worry you – you go over and over them and can't concentrate, think about, talk about much else. The worry is always on your mind. You may simultaneously be telling yourself not to think about it, but you do – and you can't stop. Like avoidance, obsessing about something is not going to make it go away. It's time to find a happy medium.

Finding your happy medium

Controlled worrying can give you a more balanced approach to your worries, where you neither obsess nor avoid the things that are troubling you.

Try this: worry time

You'll need to set aside 15 minutes.

During this time you are going to worry. You will worry as much as you like, pursue every fear, think of every little scary thing.

1 Choose a quiet time when you're unlikely to be interrupted.

2 Consider having a pen and paper to jot down notes/observations/thoughts.

3 Set an end time – it helps to have something specific to do, an appointment, a TV programme to watch, the dog to walk. Something quite 'active' (although not necessarily physical) is useful, as it will pull you out of worry time.

While you worry, try to notice what is happening: notice the four worry elements (jot them down if it helps):

1 Worried thoughts

2 Worried emotions

3 Worried body

4 Worried behaviour

Do this once a day for a minimum of two weeks, but longer if you find it helpful.

Worry time sounds grim, but studies show that it's very effective. It allows you to develop a clear perspective on your worries, instead of the usual fearful muddle. It helps you plan ways to cope and manage intrusive thoughts when they pop into your head at other times of the day (you won't think them now, you'll think them at worry time).

❝I have always been a bit of a worrier and being ill just made it a hundred times worse. I found the idea of "worry time" a bit intimidating at first. I thought my worries would get out of control. But with worry time, it's as if the worry has had its outing and I can put it away afterwards and do something I enjoy. I feel like my worrying is under control now.❞

Arthur, 56, had a perforated ulcer and haemorrhage

TIP

Ask, 'What if ...'

During worry time, as the worries flood in, you can try thinking: 'What if ...' ('OK, what if I do get ill again/have financial problems/my partner leaves me?'). 'What if ...' seems scary, but it takes away some of the power of a worry. It allows you to face it and problem solve ('OK, so if that did happen then I would do x, y and z'). Things that previously seemed unbearable might begin to feel, if not manageable, then slightly less terrifying. And you may be able to think about whether there are things you could do to try to prevent this feared event from happening in the first place.

Thinking something won't make it happen

You probably know this rationally – but even the most rational person can get surprisingly superstitious when it comes to health. This is because at times our health can feel so totally out of our control. Thoughts have a huge influence on how you feel and behave, but they cannot cause a heart attack or a recurrence of disease, or a car accident. So give yourself permission to think about the worst thing. Thinking it isn't going to make it happen.

If you don't like worry time, try this instead: the worry scale

This is slightly less intense than worry time, but still gives you some perspective on your worries. Have a scale of 1 to 10 in your head where 1 is no worries at all and 10 is total panic stations.

1 When you start to feel anxious, try to pinpoint, using your scale, how worried you are. Give the worry a score from 1–10.

2 What can you do to make the worry less of a worry?

3 If your worry is high – say a 7 or above – you could try slow breathing (page 48) or muscle squeeze–release (page 51). See if you can add in some soothing words, such as 'I am OK', 'I can do my relaxation', 'I will get through this'.

Your worry scale will help you to notice if you are getting less anxious over time; for example, a worry that was originally an 8 on your scale, may slowly become a 6 or even a 5 as you learn to cope, or do things to change it.

PANIC STATIONS

The thing to know about extreme anxiety – your level 10 – is that it can be triggered quite easily, it peaks rapidly but there is a point at which it won't get worse, and has to get better. Your fear may stay at a very high level for some time, but eventually it *will* start to drop. Psychologists in the 1950s based a phobia treatment known as 'flooding' on this fact. If someone was afraid of heights, the psychologist would do things like put them on a Ferris wheel and make it stop when their cabin reached the top. The patient would be 'flooded' with fear, but they'd have to stay at the top of the Ferris wheel until the panic subsided – and it always did. Since then, we've developed more humane treatments for phobias, but the point is: fear levels do drop. You can't stay at level 10 forever.

Tackling your worried body

The fight–flight response leaves your body in a very tense state. You therefore need to find ways to calm it down and get rid of the effects of all that adrenalin. You need to send your body signals saying, 'Turn down the volume.'

Exercising regularly, ideally outside, should be a cornerstone of your worry management. Research shows that it is a highly effective way to tackle both worried body and worried mind (see Chapter 10).

Other ways to turn down the body volume:

Slow breathing

Your first port of call when a worry kicks in is to slow your breathing down. Slowing your breathing returns your body to its pre-adrenalin balance. This sends a message to your brain saying 'the threat has gone'. The quickest, simplest and most effective way to do this is to make your out-breath longer than your in-breath. The best way to achieve this is to count.

1 As you breathe in count up to 4.

2 Hold your breath for a count of 2, and then breathe out to a count of 7.

If you prefer, breathe in for 7 and out for 11, or in for 2 and out for 8, that is fine too – the actual numbers don't matter. Just do what's comfortable, but make sure the out-breath is longer than the in-breath. And that's it: relaxation in a nutshell.

Of course, there are all sorts of embellishments and additions, but if you can crack slow breathing, you have a basic building block towards relaxation. It can help to purse your lips as you breathe out (imagine you're breathing out through a straw, blowing up a balloon or keeping a feather afloat). It also helps to pay attention to how your body feels as you breathe out: notice the way your shoulders drop, your neck muscles loosen, the tension in your chest releases. Adding a few words to yourself in your mind (calm, relax, warm, heavy, loose, smooth) can also help your body to feel that way.

❛I get tense when I notice myself struggling to balance and this makes things worse. But now I sit down, I slow down my breathing, I look out of the window to my bird table and tell myself that I am lucky to be alive. It helps.❜

Maureen, 55, had surgery for a brain aneurysm

> **TIP**
>
> ## Hi-tech help
>
> If you have a smartphone or other device, you can download podcasts and apps, and other clever things that guide you through relaxation sessions, meditations or mindfulness techniques ranging in length from a minute to an hour. These can be very helpful; however, don't get too hung up on instructions, scripts, methods or a particular voice – you don't want to be dependent on any one thing. Being able to relax yourself is an essential life skill. Like any skill, it takes practise. It is a good idea, therefore, to learn and practise some simple and solid skills when you are not in a total tizzy.

Get moving!

To burn off adrenalin you need to move your body. Vigorous movement is best, but any activity will do, even just a change of position or some stretches – whatever you can manage. This is in addition to your daily exercise routine. It is a physical way to burn off immediate worry symptoms.

> **TIP**
>
> ## Things to try
>
> Depending on your ability, obviously: go for a run, climb some stairs, do star jumps, jog on the spot, take a walk, kick a football, punch a pillow, stroll round the block, stretch, move from sofa to kitchen, walk outside to the garden, lift some weights (or even bottles of water or cans of baked beans!).

⁶⁶I was having panic attacks for about a year after my heart surgery. I can still remember; it was 15 years ago, I was sitting by the river feeling all hot and bothered and I thought, *I have got to do something about this.* So I just got up and started walking. I walked right the way past two bridges and I felt so much better. I haven't looked back, I started a local walking group for the neighbours and we've been walking ever since. ⁹

Norman, 70, had heart bypass surgery

Muscle squeeze–release

Sheila Pim's advice to the convalescents of the 1940s, in her book *Convalescence*, was to put a slow waltz on the gramophone, sit in a chair, and perform gentle arm movements before bed. The essence of this advice is delightfully sound. Before you can relax your muscles properly, you have to tense them up. Tensing and then gently releasing muscles creates a far deeper relaxation than just trying to relax them without tensing first. Even without the waltzing gramophone, this technique works. If you feel any pain at any point, stop using that muscle group.

It can help to be lying down when you first learn muscle squeeze–release. But as you get more experienced at using it, try it sitting down or even standing up. Muscle squeeze–release needs to work for you in any setting, not just when you are at home lying on your bed.

Get into a comfortable position, then:

1 Fists: clench your fists for a few seconds; feel the tension around your hands and lower arms. Release the tension and feel the relaxation flowing in.

2 Elbows: pull your elbows into your sides, hunch your shoulders around your ears, feel tightness in the muscles of your upper arms, shoulders and upper back. Hold for a few seconds and then release. Feel the tension go and the relaxation flow in.

3 Chin: pull your chin to your chest, clench your teeth and frown. This tightens the muscles of your neck and face. Focus on how hard they're working, pulling against each other, clenching tight and tense. Release and feel the muscles loosening, unwinding and becoming smooth, soft and supple.

4 Tummy: to tighten the muscles of your abdomen you can either pull your tummy in or push it out, and hold it there. Whatever you do, feel the muscles pulling tight and tense, working hard to hold the position. Then release, and feel the rush and relief of relaxation flooding in to take the place of tension.

5 Buttocks: clench your buttocks and hold. Imagine the muscles all scrunched up tight. Release and imagine the muscles smoothing out, loosening and unwinding.

6 Thighs/upper legs: do them one at a time. Lift one leg up and hold for a few seconds. Feel the muscles being pulled tight and tense. The leg may even wobble a bit. Let it down, let the tension go and feel the relief of relaxation replacing the tension. Repeat with the other leg.

7 Lower legs: you can do these at the same time. Pull your toes forward, as if towards your face, and feel the stretch in the back of your calves. Notice a gentle pulling and stretching in your lower leg and calf muscles. Imagine they are like an elastic band and, as you release, feel the tension rushing out to be replaced by relaxation.

8 Enjoy: give yourself a few moments (minutes, if you have time) to appreciate the feeling of relaxation spreading from the top of your head to the tips of your toes.

Don't get caught up in worrying that there is only one right way to do muscle squeeze–release. There isn't. It is all about tensing and then releasing your muscles. Find a way to do this that works for you.

Cool down

Physical worry symptoms – sweating, going red – can be bothersome, and make you more het up. Ways to tackle them can be very simple: splashing some water on your face, using wet wipes over your face or hands, going to a window, or outside, or even carrying a little fan around. The point is, it's worth paying attention to these things, as they all contribute to the uncomfortable feeling of being worried.

TIP

Contemplative exercise

You'll have realised, by now, that tackling worry involves both physical activity and quieter contemplation. You need to burn off that adrenalin to tackle your worried body, but you also need to tackle your worried thoughts and feelings with quieter contemplation and calming techniques. Some activities, if you are physically capable of them, are really helpful and let you do both simultaneously. Walking, swimming, yoga or gardening all fall into this category – but there are many more.
Contemplative exercise is certainly worth incorporating regularly into your life if you can.

Tackling worried thoughts

'Many patients, I find, embark on their convalescence without any clear idea of what has been happening to

> *them; what has been done for them; the whys and*
> *wherefores and what they may expect next. And with the*
> *vast majority of them, what they fear in their imaginings*
> *is far, far worse than the truth.'*

Dr George Day, 'The Tardy Convalescent'
***British Medical Journal*, 1953**

Thoughts fuel worries. A single thought can become the foundation for a positively Shard-like skyscraper of anxiety or tension. One vital way to manage anxiety, therefore, is to find ways to manage your thoughts. Thoughts are just thoughts – they are interpretations of events, not necessarily fully verified facts. One simple fact-based thought ('there's a noise') can trigger a tangle of other thoughts that may – or may not – be true ('It's a burglar!', 'Blooming neighbours!', 'What's the cat done this time?'). Often, when you worry, your thoughts race and you can become very distracted. Fortunately, there are ways to manage racing thoughts – or at the very least turn down their volume.

Thought Traps: your thoughts and why they matter

We all talk to ourselves, most of the time. There is a commentary going on inside our heads ('I did that well', 'I wish I hadn't said that', 'I must remember to . . .', 'I think he likes me'). We are so used to this commentary that most of the time we don't notice it. It is automatic, a habit. This is fine, unless for some reason we start to feel worried, scared, low or stressed. This is when those thought habits (the things you say to yourself) become stuck in harsh, unfair and unrealistic patterns.

These patterns of thinking are known as 'Thought Traps'. They can trap you into thinking, feeling and behaving in certain ways. Ways that can keep you feeling bad.

Many thoughts, however, are not facts. They are not always

a straightforward reflection of reality. They are often our own interpretations of the world. How often have you thought 'I failed that test', 'She won't call me', 'I messed up' only to discover that the actual outcome was quite different? Identifying your personal Thought Traps and building your own 'case for the defence' is a skill that takes time to develop. But it is well worth the effort. It can help you turn down the volume of your worries (stress, depression, or any other difficult emotion) dramatically. You may even be able to turn a worry off completely.

COMMON THOUGHT TRAPS

- Catastrophising: taking one fact, and jumping straight to the worst conclusion – 'I have a headache – I'm having another stroke.'

- Mind-reading: making judgements about what other people are thinking – 'They're fed up with me worrying.'

- Labelling yourself: 'I'm weak', 'I'm pathetic.'

- If ... , then ... thinking: 'If I can't stop worrying, then I'm going to get ill again.'

- Filter glasses: you only see the negatives – 'I've slipped with the diet my doctor gave me. I can't do this.'

- Fortune-telling: predicting the future – 'It's only a matter of time before I have another heart attack/stroke/car accident.'

- Shoulds and oughts: unrealistic or harsh expectations of yourself – 'I should be making the most of this valuable time, I'm lucky to be alive', 'I shouldn't worry about this silly stuff', 'My boss ought to know I'm not up to this.'

Thought Traps can really undermine our sense of who we are, influence our behaviour, damage our confidence and leave us very worried and stressed. The good news is that thoughts are just thoughts. You can question and change them. To do this you have to learn how to spot them, then remove their power.

Try this: the 'case for the defence'

First, you have to identify exactly what it is you are saying to yourself. When you feel worried, write down the actual thoughts that are going through your head. Now look closely at these thoughts. Just because they are yours, it doesn't mean you have to accept them.

Everyone deserves a good defence. You can defend yourself against your Thought Traps by questioning them, rigorously. Your 'case for the defence' will rest on three strands of argument:

1 What's the evidence?

2 Are there mitigating circumstances?

3 Is thinking like this fair or helpful?

Use this 'case for the defence' to question each Thought Trap. Here are a couple of examples:

1 Thought Trap – 'catastrophising'

Example: 'I've got a headache, it must be another stroke.'

Build your 'case for the defence':

What's the evidence? Do I have any other signs of a stroke? How similar is this to my stroke? Could there be another explanation for my headache? Have I been working at the computer without my reading glasses? Have I had headaches before that were not linked to a stroke? Am I expecting myself never to have a 'simple' headache again? What medical information do I have? Did my team tell me I might get headaches and not to worry? What did they say would cause them concern; what symptoms do I need to respond to? Do I need to act on this now or are there other steps I should try first – find my reading glasses, take a painkiller, do some relaxation?

What are the mitigating circumstances? Is anxiety playing a part here? Has my fight–flight response been set off? It is understandable that stroke is the first thing I think of after the trauma I've been through, but how similar is this situation to the one where I did have a stroke? Can I turn down the volume of my worry?

Is thinking like this fair or helpful? Is telling myself that it must be a stroke making my worry skyrocket? Is it helping me to know what to do? If I was trying to help someone else in this situation, what would I say to them to help them try to calm down and work out what to do? Can I listen to that advice myself? Let me think about the practical steps I should take now.

2 Thought Trap – shoulds and oughts

Example: 'I should be better by now.'

Build your 'case for the defence':

What's the evidence? Who says you should be better? How are you measuring better? Are you comparing yourself to one or two other people who might be quite different from you? Is there really a delay? Has your doctor told you that you should be better by now or is there actually a range of times it takes to feel better? Even if there is one area where your recovery may be slower than expected, are there other areas in which you are doing very well? If there is a genuine delay, what is your doctor's theory about why? Are they blaming you?

Mitigating circumstances Are you taking all your circumstances into account? Are there actually good reasons why this would be a slow process? Might taking your recovery slowly be the right approach for you? Have you had to cope with unexpected setbacks? Have you crumbled in the face of difficulties or setbacks or are you resiliently picking yourself up and finding ways to manage?

Is thinking like this fair or helpful? Does pressurising yourself with thoughts like this help you in your recovery process? Is comparing yourself to others fair? Is recovery a race? Are there more effective ways to motivate and encourage yourself? What are you doing well and what can you do to develop this further? Imagine if someone you love or admire was in your situation right now – would you be blaming them for not getting better quicker? Blaming yourself won't change anything. It would be far more helpful to re-channel that energy towards finding a way forward.

At first, spotting Thought Traps and providing the 'case for the defence' can feel artificial. You probably won't believe the evidence, and you'll be tempted to dismiss your mitigating circumstances or say, 'Yes it *is* fair!' But when you've done this each day for a week or two you'll stop automatically accepting your first thought. Instead, you'll 'catch it' and start to question it. This will lead to a far more balanced, calm way of thinking and this – in turn – will turn down the volume on your worries.

❝I know that when I feel achy or breathless my first thought is going to be that my heart valve is not working properly. But it is no longer my only thought. Six years on I now have the evidence to help me to distinguish between day-to-day aches and pains and anything more serious. I can now talk myself out of my immediate anxious response and take a realistic look at what is going on. I haven't had to make any trips to A&E for over three years.❞

Yvonne, 62, had aortic valve surgery

TIP

Realistic, not positive, thinking

Your 'case for the defence' is not about turning every negative thought into a positive one. You may be in a very difficult situation and trying to 'think positively' will be not only infuriating but also impossible! Instead your 'case for the defence' is about helping you to avoid falling into the trap of accepting your first (and often worst-case) scenario, allowing you to keep a balanced, realistic view and a practical approach to coping with whatever gets thrown at you.

Three quick ways to question your thoughts

1 **'Would I say this to someone I care about?'** When you spot a Thought Trap, try asking yourself, 'Would I dream of saying this to my child/best friend/spouse/sibling, if they were in a similar situation?', 'Would I train a colleague to think in this way?' It is possible to recognise the mitigating circumstances for other people, to question fairness, to

provide evidence, to accept imperfections and to allow them to learn and develop. Isn't it time to do this for yourself, too?

2 **'That's outrageous!'** We get so used to saying things to ourselves that often we don't even notice we are doing it. Another strategy, when you catch a Thought Trap, is to imagine, for a moment, that your least favourite neighbour or colleague is saying this to you ('You're weak!', 'You're a dead weight!', 'You shouldn't cry!'). Not so easy to accept, now, is it? If someone else spoke to you that way you'd probably say something like, 'That's outrageous!' and defend yourself pretty strongly. The next time you spot a Thought Trap, defend yourself ('I'm weak': 'Wait! That's an outrageous thing to say!').

3 **'Hold on ...'** If spotting thoughts, providing a 'case for the defence', and mitigating circumstances all feel too much like hard work, try just saying 'Hold on ...'. 'Hold on ...' stops a thought from getting its claws into you; for example, if you're in a 'labelling' Thought Trap ('I'm pathetic'), saying to yourself, 'Hold on ...' will force you to stop and think. If you want to, you can then question the thought.

TIP

Be the court clerk too

During your 'case for the defence' it can help to write down your answers. This will make them seem more secure, plus, you can look back later and remind yourself of more helpful and realistic responses to similar thoughts. After all, every court has to have the court clerk. Your 'case for the defence' should be no different.

How to turn down the thought volume

There are moments (waiting for test results; sitting in the doctor's waiting room) when you don't need to question worries, you simply need a short-term way to block them. 'The power of not thinking about a thing till the proper time is as useful as the power of thinking about one thing at a time', wrote Sheila Pim (*Getting Better: A Convalescent's Handbook*, 1943). These are still wise words – but how do you do this?

1 **Mental distraction** You will know what works for you – surfing the Internet, practising the guitar, doing a jigsaw puzzle, calling a friend. Mental exercises that test your powers of concentration and memory can be particularly good, as they give your brain something to do: crosswords, sudoku, learning poetry off by heart, counting back from 1,000 in threes, brain training on a games console.

2 **Writing** Jotting down worries as they pop into your mind, keeping a formal worry log book, creative writing (poetry, song lyrics, short stories, novels) can help to keep worries from escalating.

3 **Direct the thought to worry time** When that worry leaps out at you, simply say to it, 'This is not the right time. I'll see you at worry time.'

4 **Use Mindfulness** Simply acknowledge that thought, then move on. Say to yourself, 'Ah, there it is, that worry about X.' Don't judge it ('That's a horrible thought, that's awful! I mustn't think that.'). Just watch it pass through your head. When it's gone, bring yourself back – think about where you are right here and now. Try to notice: how you're breathing; the background noises; how your clothes feel on your body; what position you're in; how your tongue lies in your mouth; any smells wafting over you.

TIP
___

Be a thought detective

Taking an investigative stance can enhance the mindful approach above. Watch a worrying thought as if you're a detective doing surveillance on a suspicious character. Notice what happens to it. Does it loiter around? Does it grow bigger? Does it call in other gang members? Or does it shimmy off into the shadows? Do new thoughts come and take its place? Being a thought detective helps worries to feel less threatening. You observe them as they come and go but you don't get involved. They're just thoughts.

⦿ Before, if I stopped for some quiet time I'd end up feeling like a dam holding back a flood of thoughts. Quite often the dam would break, and I'd be overwhelmed by worries. Mindfulness has taught me to stay calm, to accept that the thoughts come, but they also go. I don't feel like a burst dam any more. I'm just an observer. ❯

Kamal, 69, had pneumonia

Lose the stiff upper lip and let it all out

Many people feel ashamed that they're getting anxious. They feel they should be 'getting back on track', 'picking up the pieces', 'being strong', 'not burdening others'. They worry that it's weak or ungrateful not to be on top form. They pretend to be 'fine and dandy'. Stiff upper lips are generally not terribly productive. Talking isn't about whingeing, or dwelling or obsessing. It is about putting things into perspective. Talking about your worries can really help to defuse them.

Your instinct is the best guide of who to talk to about this: family or friends, someone from your health-care team, someone who has been through something similar to you. Or perhaps talking to someone you don't know would work better for you: phoning a helpline, finding people to communicate with over the Internet. If you find that fear and worry are disrupting, or even dominating, your life, then talking to a therapist can help. Your doctor can advise you on this.

TIPS FOR TALKING

- Don't mind-read: you might think someone is 'too busy' to listen to your worries, or 'has enough to deal with', or 'will think I am whingeing', but this may not be true. In fact, people may be flattered, or relieved, or interested when you open up.

- Make it constructive: try to have an idea about the next step, a reward for your efforts, or perhaps just a date for when you'll talk next. It can help you to see that there is a way forward.

- Limit your talking time: therapy sessions last for 50 minutes to an hour for a reason. Both you and the person you are talking to will probably need to take a break, change the subject or go for a walk after an hour or so.

❝Even small talk can be reassuring, it takes you out of yourself, helps you to look at your situation with humour again. Once in a while I do talk to a friend about what is troubling me and it makes the world of difference. I see that he is coping, he is getting on with life and there's no reason why I can't.❞

Gavin, 57, had a heart attack

How to talk to children

When you are struggling with a health problem, it is easy to feel guilty and anxious about what all this is doing to your children (or grandchildren). You might think that the best option is to shield a child as much as possible, particularly if things are uncertain or the situation is serious. The problem is that children are awfully good at picking up on adult anxiety. If you don't keep them in the loop they tend to draw their own conclusions – and often those are even worse than the reality. If children feel there is a 'secret', they quickly feel anxious and stressed. Children also easily feel responsible when bad things happen. Your golden rules:

1 Reassure them that none of this is their fault.

2 Give them a realistic explanation of what has happened, and what is happening now.

3 Stick to normal routines as far as possible.

4 Talk to them – and allow them to ask questions. Make the conversation ongoing.

How to do this

When it comes to your children *you* are the expert. Ill health can damage your confidence. It can make you think that others – a doctor, a teacher, another family member – might be better at talking to and supporting your child than you are. This is not true. You know your child best. You may not think it right now, but you are the one who knows best how to talk to them, explore their worries and reassure them. The following strategies are some suggestions for making this work. Pick and choose: only you will know what feels appropriate to your family and your situation.

Let your child take the lead If they are asking questions, they are interested and want information. You don't necessarily have to answer all questions immediately – if you're in the fast lane of the motorway, or trying to cook dinner for ten people you may not be best placed to talk (or listen). It is OK to say something like: 'That's a really important question and I'm glad you want to talk to me. I can't really talk properly about it right now but I do want to, so can we talk when we get home/when I've done this/tonight at six?' If you do this you *must* then follow through. Set a time to talk and stick to it – don't leave it longer than 24 hours.

It's OK to show how you feel It's easy to feel guilty if you get upset in front of a child, but one vital part of parenting (or grandparenting) involves teaching children how to cope with difficult or painful emotions. If you bottle up your feelings, a child can grow up with the idea that strong feelings are bad and should be hidden. This is not in anyone's best interests. Of course, there are degrees – seeing you in extreme distress could be scary for a child – but if this does happen (and it might) be sure to explain what was going on, and talk about it later. If your child's questions or the subjects you have to talk about make you feel upset, then it's OK to let the feelings out, but be sure to find a way to calm down and move on together afterwards – something as simple as a hug and a DVD is good.

Uncertainty is OK It's tempting to think that children need certainty and facts and that if you don't know for sure it's best not to say anything. This isn't true. Most children can cope with some uncertainty. It is much harder for children to think that information is being hidden from them. It isn't easy to tell your child that you aren't sure what the future holds, but you can explain what might happen, and then keep them involved and updated. After a conversation like this, check that they are OK with what you've told them. Ask if they need any more information. Then keep the lines of communication open.

Use resources Your doctor, nurse, physiotherapist, or another health professional, may be able to advise you on simple, child-friendly ways to describe what has happened to you. Health charities often have useful leaflets written specifically for children. You could also try your library or bookshop.

Keep to normal routines There will inevitably be some disruption, but try to keep your child's life as 'normal' as possible. Maintain the usual activities, chores, rules as far as you can. This is their anchor. You might be tempted not to bother with bedtimes or table manners, to throw homework out the window and shower your child with attention and treats. Although this is entirely appropriate during an immediate crisis, it is less helpful afterwards. In fact, it signals to a child that the crisis is still very close – and their world might be disrupted at any moment. Resuming normal routines sends the message that the world is safe and secure again.

Give them a supporting role Obviously, this is age and circumstance dependent, but in general, far from feeling burdened, most children will feel included and engaged if they can help you. Talk to them about things they can do; you could have some ideas up your sleeve in case they have none. Could they be your exercise buddy, smoothie maker, relaxation instructor, foot-massager? Don't pressurise, but if your child goes out of their way to help or support you, make sure to comment on it, and thank them.

Child carers

If your child is your main carer, it is vital to find support for them (and for yourself). Talk to your health-care team about your circumstances; be completely honest – none of this is your fault, and getting help is the best thing you can possibly do for your child. It is also a good idea to contact a young carers organisation (see Resources) for ideas, advice and support.

TIP

Keep on talking

The one big heart-to-heart talk is great, but it is not enough. You may need to repeat things many times, to give regular updates and to review what's happened. If the chance to talk never seems to pop up spontaneously, you might consider a weekly family meeting where you all talk about what's been going on for you this week. Finally, if you feel your child needs some extra help in coping – and many children do – then talk to your GP. There will be local services to support families in situations like yours.

Your health problem is very likely to disrupt your child's life, but it does not have to be damaging. Indeed, handled well and with the right support, such challenges can be emotionally strengthening for a child. Don't let your fear, guilt or loss of confidence drive a wedge between you. You are still the parent – and parenting is about so much more than physical abilities. You can all come through this stronger than ever.

* * * * *

Tackling your worries may seem complicated, but really it's quite simple. There is probably a time and place for that old-time medicinal snifter, but in general worry management is not about temporary blotting out. It's about systematic, calm defusing. When you boil it down, worry management is just a question of understanding how worries work, then learning simple tricks for turning the volume down.

You'll get better and better at this the more you do it. Worry management is a skill, like bricklaying, bookkeeping or brain surgery. You have to learn it and practise it until you get really good at it. When you do, you will find that you are no longer ruled by your worries, crippled by anxiety or paralysed by fears. Your worries probably won't vanish completely, but they will be under control. Then you can get on with the real business of recovery.

NOTES FOR CARERS

'Apprehension, uncertainty, waiting, expectation, fear of surprise do a patient more harm than any exertion. Remember, he is face to face with his enemy all the time, internally wrestling with him, having long internal conversations with him.'

Florence Nightingale, *Notes on Nursing*, **1859**

Caring for someone who is 'internally wrestling' with their demons is not an easy task. You probably have some internal wrestling matches going on yourself. You too have been through the mill. You may have huge worries of your own. You may be putting on a brave face in order to be strong, but this does not lessen the pressure you are under. Here are some ways to manage your own worries:

1 **Understand what's worrying you**, and use the coping strategies. Read this chapter, and think about how it applies to you, rather than the person you are caring for. You need to find ways to 'turn down the volume' of your own worries. Key strategies include: worry time (page 45), relaxation techniques (page 51), and tackling your Thought Traps (page 54). You will be better able to care for your loved one if you are not sapped by your own worries. You may also see which

strategies work well, and encourage the person you are caring for to use them too.

2 **Accept that some worry is inevitable** Worry is a natural consequence of a health crisis, and it is going to take time for you all to feel calm again. You need to learn which of your loved one's physical sensations need medical attention, and which are the normal aches and pains of day-to-day life. It is important for you to be just as clear about this as your loved one. If you're uncertain, you may find yourself worrying about things that are perfectly fine – and that's exhausting.

3 **Set limits** It is good to talk about your loved one's worries, but this can become overwhelming. Make it a rule not to talk about a particular worry for more than about half an hour at a time – at the most. It is important to find a balance between helpful sharing, and getting caught up in a spiral of unresolved fears. Remember, too, that you do not always have to talk about a worry the moment it rears its head. If you are in the middle of something, or not in a listening frame of mind, then it is perfectly OK to say that you can't talk right now – but then to arrange (and keep) a time when you will talk about it.

4 **Try not to dismiss their worry** with comments like 'That's silly' or 'Don't think like that' or 'You'll be fine.' This sort of comment generally doesn't stop someone from worrying. In fact, it can actually make them feel even more worried as they start to feel they are not coping. Remember that you do not have to solve the worry for them.

Instead, remind them of their worry-management strategies: slow breathing, muscle squeeze–release, writing the worry down, catching their Thought Traps. Practical suggestions can be far more helpful than saying 'Don't worry!'

5 **Seek help** If your life is dominated by worry, if the worry (theirs or yours) stops you from getting on with life, or if you find you are avoiding things you'd like to do, then talk to your doctor. Your doctor or someone from your loved one's medical team will be used to talking about worry after illness or injury. They should be able to advise you on how to find the support you need.

❝I work in a GP practice and after my husband had his aneurism he would come to pick me up from work and get his blood pressure checked every day. That was fine for a few weeks but he got really upset one day when a nurse said she was too busy to check it. When he calmed down we both realised we needed to find other ways to put his mind at rest. He agreed to cut down how often he came to my work, and over time he has learnt to use relaxation or go for a walk when he feels himself getting wound up.❞

**Julie, 53, wife of Mark, 52, who had
surgery for an aortic aneurism**

THREE

RUSSIAN GYMNASTICS

COPING WITH STRESS

In Russia in the 1920s, exhausted workers were bundled off for a fortnight a year to 'Houses of Rest' where they were put through a doctor-led programme of hydrotherapy (including douches, baths and dips in 'open waters') to improve their metabolism, 'rebalance' their energy, and establish 'normal blood circulation'. Gymnastics were deemed 'most essential' in the House of Rest, as were 'lessons in the art of resting'.

Ill-health – and its aftermath – is a lot like hard labour. It can be stressful, relentless and exhausting. A Russian gymnastics regime may not be the answer, but the ideas behind that House of Rest are surprisingly spot-on even today. Nobody is going to insist that you leap from the vaulting horse into the village pond, or start douching in freezing water six times a day; however, this chapter will give you some key strategies for coping with the inevitable stresses and strains that ill-health can bring.

What is stress?

It sounds like a silly question, but stress is actually surprisingly difficult to define. One person's stress is another person's excitement. You might hear a teenager say, 'Oh my God, I'm so stressed, I don't know what to wear to the party tonight.' But the same word – stress – is used to describe what a soldier experiences in battle. There is no blood test or scan that can identify stress. It is an internal, personal, psychological experience.

Essentially, stress is about *overload*. Unhelpful stress kicks in when you *perceive* (that is, you think or believe) that you do not have the capacity to manage the demands you are facing.

How you perceive your abilities can change day to day. On some days you might be able to cope with anything, but on others the same events would completely stress you out. Perhaps you woke up feeling tired, or you have a headache or have been busy for days – for whatever reason, you just don't feel as strong and capable as usual. Stress starts to build.

Spotting the signs of stress

Some of the signs will be obvious to you, but others might be far more subtle. It is worth understanding exactly how stress manifests itself for you. You might be surprised by what you uncover. Common signs of stress are:

Thinking signs Short-term memory problems; difficulty concentrating; racing, intrusive, unhelpful thoughts; decision-making difficulties; inability to 'switch off'; thoughts that focus on what you cannot do or how much there is left to do; loss of confidence in your ability to achieve what you want to achieve.

Feeling signs Feeling tense; agitated; irritable; sad; depressed; lonely; overloaded; overwhelmed; helpless.

Physical signs Having tight muscles; aching muscles; headaches; altered breathing patterns; increased heart rate; tightness/butterflies in the tummy; stomach aches; nausea; tiredness.

Behaviour signs Being snappy and irritable; experiencing appetite changes; sleep problems; less energy and activity; seeing other people less; eating; drinking (alcohol) or smoking more.

The stress tipping point

Often, when people are stressed they say that something 'tipped me over the edge'. A certain amount of stress can actually be useful – it can be a great motivator, helping you perform brilliantly in a job interview, revise for an exam, or talk to the bank manager. Life would be pretty dull without a bit of stress.

The trouble is that stress does not arrive in neat packages at just the right time to ensure that we reach our full potential. It can land on you in great big wallops.

&My husband was diagnosed with dementia, we were moving house and I had my stroke all in a single fortnight. I felt like my world had fallen apart. 9

Elaine, 72, had a stroke

When stress involves such feelings of major overload it is no longer positive or motivating. You don't feel 'buzzy' and powerful, you feel tense, inefficient, unhappy, wound up or overwhelmed. You feel you've been pushed over the edge.

A health problem can do this very effectively. Psychologists have developed a stress scale of 43 particularly stressful circumstances. Number one on the list is the death of a spouse, closely followed by divorce. Personal illness or injury comes in at number six.

Why do health problems make you stressed?

There is often pressure – either self-imposed or from others – to look and sound as if you are doing brilliantly. You're supposed to look just as good, if not better than before. You're supposed to feel optimistic. Your stiff upper lip must be made of reinforced steel. If, deep down, you do not feel either strong or confident, then these expectations can add to your stress.

‶I felt it was vital to put on a good show for the family, for my children and in particular my elderly parents. I didn't want to burden any of them with the idea that I might be finding life difficult after getting back from hospital. I also thought that if I could pretend to other people that I felt this way, maybe I'd start believing it myself. It didn't work. I ended up taking on far too much, not asking for help. Soon I stopped sleeping. It was only after I caught another chest infection and nearly ended up back in hospital that I realised I had to do things differently.″

**Hannah, 47, had pneumonia and
spent ten days in intensive care**

You may also be facing ongoing health issues, having to learn new skills (or re-learn old skills), absorb new information, follow medical regimes, rebuild your strength, communicate effectively, get to know the new you – develop your 'new normal'. There may also be a build-up of tasks from when you were out of action. If you feel you can't meet all of these demands, your stress levels rocket.

Is stress bad for you?

'Stress is the top cause of workplace sickness', 'Is stress ageing you by a decade?', 'Cop job stress made me forget my family', 'Xmas shopping stress can kill you', 'Is stress killing us all?', 'Stress of 21st century puts Britons at greater risk of stroke', 'Stress fed my cancer', 'Prolonged stress can shrink the brain', 'Stress is the Black Death of the 21st century'.

These are just a handful of stress-related headlines from a couple of Britain's best-selling newspapers. If you believe the media, stress causes cancer, heart disease, stroke, infections, accidents and any number of other health horrors. You name it, stress is to blame.

The medical reality – based on scientific fact – paints a far less dramatic picture.

According to the British Heart Foundation, stress is not a direct risk factor for cardiovascular disease. According to Macmillan Cancer Support there is no evidence that stress causes cancer or affects its growth. These statements might not make newspaper-flogging headlines, but they are based on the most up-to-date and large-scale medical research studies.

Yes, stress makes you feel rotten. It may even have an impact on your immune system, making you more vulnerable to coughs, colds and other illnesses. It can also slow the body's healing process. Research into stress and illness is very complicated, but large-scale, high-quality studies do not show that stress itself directly causes serious illnesses such as cancer or heart attack; however there *is* a lot of research showing that the unhelpful and unhealthy ways in which we respond to stress can make us seriously ill.

The evidence, when it comes to major health problems like cancer, heart disease and stroke, is that if you respond to stress by smoking, drinking alcohol, over-eating, not exercising, ignoring early warning signs or withdrawing from your friends and family, then you increase your risk of ill-health. If, on the other hand, you respond to stress by finding helpful, health-promoting ways to cope (which frankly work a lot better anyway), then being stressed is not a health risk.

> Stress, itself, does not seriously harm your health, but how you respond to it might.

Of course, there is a vicious circle here too. Every time you stumble across another silly and ill-informed newspaper article saying that stress is killing you, you feel even more tense. Worrying about what stress is doing to your body can, in itself, be hugely stressful.

Stress management strategies

The key to stress management is to crack the vicious circle by learning simple, healthy and effective ways to cope.

Try this: keep a stress record

Keeping a stress record for two weeks will give you a lot of useful information. It will help you to identify and understand the following:

1 What, exactly, makes you stressed (you might think it's obvious, but by doing this, you'll probably uncover that unexpected things push you over the edge too).

2 How you respond, physically and emotionally, when stressed.

Getting to know your stress is the first vital step towards managing it. Twice a day – for example, before lunch and before going to bed – write down how stressed you felt during that portion of the day. Use a scale of 0–5 (0 = no stress and 5 = extremely stressed). If you have given yourself a 3 or more, it is time to take a closer look. See if you can:

1 **Identify the trigger/tipping point** What pushed you over the edge? Was it a specific event (your boss giving you a new task, a friend's unhelpful comment, another bill arriving)? Or is it more internal (a headache, just feeling down, the fear of a follow-up appointment, the thought that you have too much to do, the idea that you did something badly)?

2 **Identify what happened when you became stressed** Did you feel physical tension, have racing thoughts, feel butterflies in your tummy, snap at the next person who spoke to you (or all of the above)?

3 **Identify anything you did to manage your stress** Did you breathe deeply, ask for help, try to do ten things at once, cancel fun things, order a takeaway, reach for a glass of whisky? Rate your stress management strategy on a scale of 0–5 (0 = as well as possible and 5 = as badly as possible).

TIP

Don't stop if it's helpful

An ongoing stress record will give you a way to monitor your stress levels and will also help you to notice when they start to reduce. This can be great motivation to continue your stress-reducing strategies.

❝I felt incredibly stressed when I came out of hospital. Monitoring my stress helped me to recognise that I dreaded mornings and evenings because I found dressing and undressing so difficult and stressful. Eventually I spoke to an occupational therapist who told me about "grab-it-sticks" to help you with your knickers and tights. I still cry with laughter when I think of myself manoeuvring the stick, my knickers and my body. But it was wonderful, because at last I knew what to do and felt I could cope.❞

Janice, 48, had a hip replacement

Anger

Your life has been turned upside down. You have faced threats and danger. You have had to allow others to take control – maybe you've even had to 'put your life in their hands'. You've been through pain and any number of other physical discomforts and indignities. Your future might feel uncertain. Maybe you've had angry thoughts like, 'Why me?', 'Why now?', 'If only . . .' or 'It's not fair.' If so, you are far from alone. It is perfectly reasonable to feel angry when your health is under threat. Anger, in this situation, is normal.

Anger is not always a bad or dangerous emotion. It is a natural part of your instinctive 'fight or flight' response (yes, it's the 'fight' part – see page 38). Although fisticuffs are rarely helpful, some people do manage to channel their 'revved up' angry feelings into constructive behaviour.

❝My heart attack at the age of 27 just felt so unfair. All my friends were fit and active and I had been too – I was actually in the gym when it happened. For a few weeks I thought my life was over. Then the anger kicked in, and I realised that I wasn't going to let this disease beat me. I started to build up my strength again, and every time I went to the gym it felt like I was actively fighting my disease – I was getting my own back on it.❞

Adam, 30, had a heart attack

Anger, however, becomes problematic when it makes you see threats and wrongdoing where none exist, and when it has an impact on your life – or on other people. If you are already feeling stressed and overloaded – and that can go with the territory after a health crisis – this becomes more likely.

Other than the obvious loss of control, and a sense of unfairness or 'wrongness', you are also coping with expectations about your recovery. If you expected to be 'bouncing back' (or at least feeling better than this by now), but you aren't, you may have huge feelings of disappointment, fear or worry. This, too, can make you angry.

Sometimes the anger is obviously connected to what happened.

❝I never thought I would be like this a whole year after the accident, when the original injury wasn't really that extreme. I just don't feel I've recovered – I'm back cycling again, but I still have low-level back pain. I've become totally irrational towards car drivers. I think I must be channelling all my anger on to them. I've got myself into more than one road-rage incident when people cut me up – and a couple of times it's got quite nasty. I know this isn't helping anything, but there's nothing I can do – I just see red.❞

Claudia, 33, suffered severe cuts, bruising and a broken jaw when knocked off her bicycle

Sometimes anger can show itself indirectly – you may, for example, become enraged at something seemingly small or tangential, and not really know why. Your anger might be focused on one person, or situation, when really it's about something much wider.

Anger can easily dominate and become destructive. But there are many very effective ways to defuse it. Here are your main strategies:

Recognise your anger

Anger, either verbal or physical, can explode with little warning. It may feel like it happens out of the blue, but that is rarely the case. Usually there are thoughts, feelings or physical tensions simmering away underneath the surface – and then they blow. You can't tackle this unless you recognise it. Your best approach is to use the stress-management strategies in this chapter to pin down your angry thoughts, angry feelings and angry behaviour. Try to work out what triggers your anger and what happens to your mind and body when you get angry. You can then try to manage the underlying tensions – stresses, fears and frustrations.

Above all, it helps simply to be aware of the complex factors that are intimately bound up in any angry outbursts you're having.

Use anger-management tactics

Avoid your 'triggers' This is the one time when avoidance can be helpful! Try to work out what tends to trigger your outbursts, then – if possible – find ways to avoid these triggers. It could be something relatively simple like changing your route to avoid getting stuck in traffic. Or it could be a more complex change such as reducing (or even stopping) your contact with people who trigger your anger. These changes can be temporary. Anger tends to come in waves. If you are in a particularly stressful situation at the moment, giving yourself a break from situations that you know will wind you up might be enough to get you to a calmer state.

Watch out for Thought Traps Expectations (directed towards yourself or others) can make you angry, if they aren't met. If your thoughts are full of 'should', 'must', 'have to', 'never' (for example, 'I should be able to walk without pain by now') these thoughts need tackling. Mind-reading is also a potent anger fuel ('He just isn't bothered', 'She doesn't want me here'). Try to identify your Thought Traps and then build your case for the defence: look at the evidence ('Why should I be able to walk without pain? Did the doctor tell me this specifically? Or are there, in fact, a variety of time frames for recovery?'). Make sure you consider the mitigating circumstances ('I had that fall – it has delayed my recovery'). And ask if it's fair or helpful to think this way: could you find a more realistic, kind way to talk to yourself?

Try this: bomb disposal

Aim to defuse your anger bomb before it blows. To do this, try to identify what happens to you before you blow: do you grind your teeth, clench your fists, breathe fast, feel hot, start to feel shaky? This is your burning fuse. The trick is to identify it, then find ways to release the physical tension before it takes over and you explode. A bout of physical exercise (if you are up to it) or a muscle squeeze–release (see page 51) are ideal bomb-disposal strategies. Or try: punching a pillow; kicking a ball against a wall; shouting (ideally in an empty room) – or basically anything that leaves you feeling warm, tired, spent. Quieter strategies also work. Try: slow and belly breathing (pages 48 and 92); splashing your face with cold water; spraying your favourite perfume onto your neck and wrists (this can become a cue to calm down). You may have to experiment and find what works best for you.

TIP

Express your anger – safely

We are often scared of anger and so we work hard to suppress it. But, like all other emotions, suppression is usually only a temporary fix. Talking about your anger can help; however, if a person is triggering your anger, you need to think carefully about whether it's likely to be best to talk to them directly or to someone else – a friend or counsellor.

Try this: let it go

The 'let it go' tactic (page 83) is particularly useful for anger. When someone is winding you up, try to say to yourself: 'Let it go', 'This isn't really about me', 'This is old news', 'I can move on.' Anger can make situations seem very personal. It can reopen old wounds. But there is a lot you can do to stop this happening and therefore prevent a situation from escalating. This simple strategy can work wonders.

Try this: the empty chair

First, make sure you are alone! Then, imagine that the person or source of your anger (perhaps the illness or injury itself) is sitting in the chair opposite you.

1 Now let rip – say (or scream or shout) everything you need to say. You don't have to be reasonable or balanced – just let the fury burst out. This may sound insane, but it can be a huge source of relief for many people.

2 Express your anger creatively: turn it into song lyrics, poetry, art, pottery, craft – anything. If creativity is your thing, this can be a big release.

3 Write it down. Keep an anger diary (under lock and key!), and at the end of the day write down those things that are making you angry. Alternatively, write – but *don't ever post* – a furious letter to the person/source of your anger. Be as livid, embittered and vile as you want to – no holds barred. Just get it all out. When you've read or reread your letter, tear it into tiny pieces or burn it on the fire and watch the paper – and your anger – disperse.

Get help If you feel that your anger is dominating your life, or that you 'medicate' it with cake, cigarettes, alcohol or drugs, or if your anger is reaching a point where you risk hurting yourself or others, it is time to get professional help from a counsellor or trained anger-management therapist. Start by talking to your GP. Doing this is wise and sensible. Anger is nothing to be ashamed of. It's a perfectly understandable and normal response to what you've been through. Don't struggle on alone.

> **TIP**
>
> ### Let it go and forgive
>
> Holding on to anger and resentment is a bit like drinking poison and expecting the other person to die. It can be deeply self destructive. Sometimes the best thing to do is lower your standards and move on. When you find yourself getting wound up by someone's perceived inadequacies, ask yourself these two important questions:
>
> * Can I let it go?
> * Can I forgive them?
>
> If you can do this, your anger will diminish considerably.

❝At the beginning of my recovery my poor husband couldn't do anything right. If I asked him to buy orange juice he came back from the shop with orange squash instead of fresh juice. When I asked for toast for breakfast, he gave me a piece of carbon. He got cross, I got cross – it was so stressful. I consciously made myself appreciate his position, lower my expectations and instead recognise his efforts. It worked – most of the time!❞

Marina, 55, had a hysterectomy

What to do about stress

Now you have identified how your particular stress works, it's time to tackle it. The five keys to managing stress are:

1 Time management

2 Communication

3 Tackling your stressed body

4 Tackling your stressed thoughts

5 Learning relaxation techniques

Time management

It is very common to get to the point where you think 'there just aren't enough hours in the day to get everything done'. This time-pressure can make you rush around like a lunatic. You try to get everything done but do nothing properly, or you stall completely. Everything seems impossible, you feel lethargic, stuck and even more overloaded.

Time management might sound very officey, but it is a brilliant stress-busting tool. In essence it just means prioritising and planning so that the mass of crazy, impossible demands become something more organised and manageable.

The three golden rules of time management

1 **Do one thing at a time** (starting with the most urgent and important). You may be the world's greatest multi-tasker, but when you're stressed, trying to do several things at once is only going to overload you even more. You may have to stop one task in order to focus on a new, even more important and urgent task that has cropped up, but this is better than trying to do everything at once. This is actually incredibly hard to do. Your instinct will probably be, 'I have to! There's no time!' But try to force yourself to stop. You will soon find that you are more efficient, and calm, if you tackle things one at a time. You may even find you get more done.

2 **Take breaks** When you are stressed it is easy to 'push on through' – plough on to the wee small hours, miss meals, survive on energy drinks and black coffee – pushing through until the task is complete. Instead, try to take constructive

breaks (even as short as 10 minutes is worth it) to do something restorative.

3 **Manage your expectations** The list of tasks will, in fact, never end. The idea that you'll finish the day with your to-do list done and your in-tray empty is, sadly, a fantasy; however, if you can finish your day with the urgent and key tasks completed, or at least on track, and with a plan for what needs doing the next day, this is a huge achievement. It will go a long way towards reducing your stress.

❛I was running a small landscape gardening company and had recently started a degree in business as I was planning to expand the company, when I was diagnosed with bowel cancer. I went back to work a few weeks after my treatment ended and although I could just about keep my head above water with the business itself, the degree was just too much. I was too exhausted to study in the evenings, and the stress built up. Once I took the decision not to do it, I felt so much better – the stress lifted, I felt I could breathe again. Even though the college would only refund half my course fee, it was worth it.❜

Nick, 49, had bowel cancer

Try this: rate your tasks

This is a way to clear a space in your brain. It will give your overloaded mind some perspective and can also help you work out, on a more practical level, what needs to be done and how to do it.

Write a list of all the demands/tasks/activities you are expecting yourself to do (or that others are expecting from you). Now, work out which tasks:

• are very important and urgent (they have to be done, and soon),

- are important but less urgent (could they be delayed?),
- are less important and less urgent (could they be dropped?).

You could also put a note next to each task to show whether it's something you could get help with.

You may need to take this a step further, and plan exactly how you are going to get these tasks done – and by which date. To do this you could simply schedule them in a diary. Or you could write a more detailed daily, and weekly, plan.

Communicate about your stress

After illness or injury it can be very hard to negotiate about what you can or cannot take on. You may be in a state of flux, physically, practically and emotionally. You, yourself, might not know what you are capable of yet – and if you don't know, then how is a spouse, partner, friend or colleague supposed to know? You may also feel under considerable pressure to 'bounce back' enthusiastically. It is easy to end up with the feeling that you are failing, or not doing things properly, or 'letting people down'. It is vital, therefore, to learn to ask for help and to say no and to communicate clearly with people about why you are doing so.

> ❝I have always looked after my grandchildren after school, but after my heart attack I didn't feel up to doing it every day. Eventually, I explained to my daughter that I still wanted to be involved but couldn't manage every day. She agreed – she felt I was still supporting her, and the last thing she wanted was to overload me.❞
>
> **Christine, 63, had a heart attack**

When communicating about your stress remember:

- Be clear. State your needs and be clear about your abilities. This is not a sign of weakness, it is a key assertiveness skill.

It helps to clarify the situation so that you can come up with a workable solution.

- Accept that it is OK – sometimes essential – to ask for help.

- Accept that it is OK – sometimes essential – to say no.

- Recognise that any changes may be temporary – this is a fluid process, and you can frequently review it to see what your needs are now.

- Don't expect other people to mind-read: nobody can magically know what you think or feel, or what you can do, unless you tell them (calmly).

- Show your appreciation – it actually feels good to appreciate others, and this can reduce your stress as well as boost them.

How to tackle your stressed body

It is easy to slip into unhealthy habits when stressed – eating too much, or the wrong thing, or too little, drinking too much alcohol, not exercising, smoking, staying up late or getting up early. In the short term, these things might seem like good stress relievers, but they only store up problems. It is also tempting when stressed to skip the rehab exercises, dietary changes or follow-up appointment. These are the very behaviours that make stress damaging to your health.

❝When I came out of hospital, the demands of being a single mum just felt overwhelming. I knew I shouldn't, but I went back to smoking and having a couple of drinks at the end of each day. I didn't follow the diet I was supposed to follow. I just felt so wound up and didn't know any other way to unwind.❞

Joanne, 38, had septicaemia

Tackling unhelpful habits can feel like just another stress. How on earth are you going to quit smoking or drinking, or start jogging, or find time for – for goodness sake! – bubble baths and meditation? That's just not going to happen!

You're right. This is completely fair enough. Instead of thinking that you need a total lifestyle and body overhaul, and knowing there's no way you can possibly do this, try to tackle just one thing. Find something you do when stressed that you know is not helpful. Just one. *That's* the thing you are going to focus on.

You may be spoilt for choice here. A good way to identify which behaviour to tackle first is to ask your doctor which change would have the biggest positive impact on your health (or which is the most achievable for you, given your health). Taking just one step towards healthier stress management will boost your confidence. It will show you that change is possible. Slowly, you can start to tackle your other habits. Your stress will diminish more gradually but you'll get there – and getting there is the most important thing.

TIP

Switch your props

You may be using unhealthy behaviours as 'props' – that is, ways to get through the stress. Try to think about things you can do to unwind beyond booze, chocolate, cigarettes or whatever your unhealthy 'props' may be. Simple things like a favourite film, a glass of sparkling water with ice and lemon, a walk in the park, an afternoon's fishing or watching cricket, a long hot bath, a delicious fruit salad (prepared in advance) or a chat to a good friend may actually be very effective stress-releasers.

See if you can replace your unhealthy habits with any of these healthier behaviours.

Get moving!

Exercise is an essential part of stress management – it releases endorphins (the body's feel-good chemicals), improves low mood, increases energy levels, promotes good sleep and increases your confidence. All of this is extremely effective at managing stress. But there is more. Exercise increases the blood flow around your body, including the blood flow to your brain. When you are stressed, your brain is very busy – there are thoughts, worries and plans rushing around it all the time. This process actually builds up toxic waste products in your brain that can cause that cotton-wool feeling – where you 'can't think straight'. Improving the blood flow to your brain – by getting some exercise – helps clear these waste products faster. In other words, a walk round the block can – quite literally – clear your head. For more on exercise – how, how much and when – see Chapter 10.

Tackle your stressed thoughts

Our stress is defined by how we see the demands we are facing. This doesn't mean we can simply think the stress away – the psychiatrists' stress scale (page 73) shows that some events are inherently 'stressful'; however, it is very clear that how we think about the demands we face has a huge effect on how stressed we feel.

Common stress Thought Traps

- Unrealistic expectations: 'I should be able to manage this myself', 'I must not ask for help', 'I ought to be doing as much as I did before I was ill.'

- Filter glasses: 'I haven't achieved anything today', 'I can't cope', 'I'm useless.'

- Minimising: 'I managed to do some work, but the quality was awful', 'I went to an exercise class but I was the worst in the group', 'I crossed a couple of items off my to-do list but there are four new items on it already.'

- Catastrophising: 'I'll never get this all done', 'I'll always be stuck like this, there is no way out', 'I had a cigarette last night – I've failed', 'There is nothing I can do, I'm going to get more and more stressed, and this is going to cause terrible damage', 'If I don't sort this out now I'll lose my job/my relationship/my future.'

- Mind-reading: 'He/she can see I am not coping', 'No one wants to help me sort out my stress', 'They will want to get rid of me if I tell them I am stressed.'

Build your 'case for the defence'

Once again, you're going to be your own defence lawyer. So, when you spot these stress Thought Traps, ask yourself:

What is the evidence? Have you got through the day having achieved absolutely nothing? You might not think what you've done is particularly valuable or that it's not enough ('OK, so I walked to the post box – but I used to run marathons and I still have so much admin to do'). This does not wipe out what you *have* done. Are you prioritising and managing your essential tasks? You could try writing a 'have done' list, where you jot down even the smallest things you managed today. Ask yourself if other people are really expecting you to do all of this without some help. It's surely possible that those around you might want to support you if they can. Saying no does not mean that you are rejecting someone. You could try to think of other ways of explaining why you can't do what they are asking of you.

What are the mitigating circumstances? Your health has been shaken. You have faced all sorts of physical and mental challenges. You physically cannot do as much as you managed before. Tasks will build up. This is why you are struggling. Nobody is suggesting you give up trying, but instead of beating yourself up about what you can't do, try to measure your achievements against yesterday or last week's scale, not your pre-illness or injury levels. Try to identify the effort involved rather than the result. Yes, a trip to the post box seems trivial – it used to be a doddle, but if it now requires a huge mental and physical effort then it is a big achievement. You did it. This is progress. And when you are trying to get better and manage your stress, any progress is good news.

Is thinking like this fair or helpful? Expecting yourself to instantly 'bounce back' is not fair. Making comparisons to how you were previously is harsh and unhelpful. So is thinking that there is no way through this stress. Think about how you have managed stressful situations in the past. Ask yourself whether those situations lasted forever. Telling yourself that you are hopeless, weak, overloaded, stuck and unable to cope will only add to your stress. Far from motivating you to do more, these thoughts leave you feeling less able to manage. This is when the 'vicious circle' of stress kicks in.

Ask yourself what you would do if someone you do not like or respect started saying to you, 'You're rubbish! You'll never manage all of this!' Would you simply nod your head and agree with them? Unlikely. Although you might acknowledge that the situation is tough, you'd also probably point out that you're up to it; you might mention things you've already achieved; you might tell them how you plan to tackle the challenges ahead. We say things to ourselves that we would not dream of letting other people say to us. That's just not fair or helpful.

Relax . . .

> ❛My wife won't let me drive, answer the phone, open the door, make a sandwich, even get myself a cup of tea, she is constantly telling me to relax. I know this is her way of caring for me, but the truth is the more she does for me the more she takes away what I can do. So when she is telling me to sit down, relax and have a cup of tea, it makes me really stressed.❜
>
> **David, 69, had bronchial pneumonia**

If you're being told to relax, you may already be in a white-knuckled state: waiting for test results, undergoing an unpleasant medical procedure, feeling overloaded, trying to hold your tongue. You wouldn't have time for an aromatherapy massage even if you had the inclination. Relax? No chance.

There are several quick strategies that every stressed person should know about. In fact they should be handed out on prescription to anyone who has ever had health problems. These simple techniques are proven to reduce immediate stress: they slow rapid, shallow breathing and loosen tight, tense, aching muscles. You may think you don't need this sort of thing. But if you resort to telling yourself to relax – or worse, having someone else bark the word at you – then the opposite is likely to happen.

Try this: quick fix – belly breathing

When stressed, your breathing becomes rapid and shallow. This physical response actually keeps you stressed. Belly breathing reverses this – and is therefore calming.

1 Sit in a comfortable position (although you could stand or, ideally, lie down).

2 Put one hand on your chest and the other on your tummy just around or below your belly button.

3 Take a deep breath in through your nose. As you breathe in, try to make the hand on your tummy come out further than the hand on your chest.

4 Now breathe out slowly through your mouth. As you breathe out, imagine that the hand on your tummy is pushing the air out of your body – get the tummy hand to move further in than the hand on your chest. This full out-breath will properly empty your lungs. They will be more able to fill up properly with the next in-breath.

5 Repeat 2–3 times. Try to concentrate on how this deep abdominal breathing makes you feel. See if you can notice your shoulders dropping and your muscles loosening as relaxation flows through your body.

For an alternative quick fix you could also try slow breathing (Chapter 2, page 48). It's always good to have a couple of tricks up your sleeve.

Try this: slow fix – mindfulness

Mindfulness is a major new approach in psychology that has its origins in Buddhist meditation. It is a longer-term approach to managing stress, but it isn't complicated, and scientific studies show that it is highly effective for dealing with stress. It's hard to describe mindfulness meaningfully in a paragraph – ideally you want to go on a course (or at the very least read a book: try *Mindfulness: A Practical Guide to Finding Peace in a Frantic World* by Mark Williams and Danny Penman). Don't let this put you off though. Anyone can benefit from mindfulness.

In essence, mindfulness helps you learn to be aware of your situation, and to observe yourself – without making any judgements. This helps you to break unhelpful and stressful patterns of thinking, feeling and behaving. It's easy to think constantly about the past or future and miss out on the present. Mindfulness helps you to be more in the present – and this, in turn, reduces stress (think about how much time you spend being stressed and worried about what has happened in the past, or what's going to happen next).

A MINDFUL MEDITATION

This exercise will give you a flavour of what mindfulness is about.

1 Set a timer for 3 minutes – ideally something with a gentle 'wake-up' noise rather than a blaring alarm.

2 Sit on a chair, feet firmly on the ground, back straight and ideally not leaning on the back of the chair, so you are awake and alert.

3 Close your eyes. Notice your breath in and then your breath out – there is no right or wrong way to breathe in this exercise, just notice what you feel as you breathe in and then out.

4 Your mind will wander. When thoughts appear, instead of trying to examine them, solve them, or get rid of them – simply notice them happening. You could say to yourself, for example, 'Ah yes, I am planning/reviewing/dreaming/worrying.' Then bring your mind back to your breath again and the sensations you notice (your body on the chair, feet on the ground, breeze on your face, and so on).

5 Keep doing this until it's time to open your eyes.

Over time and with practise this simple meditation allows you to observe your thoughts but to stop struggling with them. They just come and go. They're just thoughts. You realise, eventually, that you are not your thoughts. This realisation is profoundly liberating. It can help enormously with stressful situations. The aim is to do a meditation like this most days. The best way is to settle on a time of day (first thing in the morning or before bed are good times) and make it into a habit. Schedule it, if that helps.

Develop stress busters

It can, of course, be incredibly hard to find time to unwind. Timetabling some healthy, de-stressing activities into your week or day makes them far more likely to happen. This is not another exercise that requires you to rethink your life. All you have to do is identify what helps you to unwind and then do it (unless it is the packet of cigarettes, glass of gin or large portions of chicken tikka masala. In which case, turn back to page 88 to think about how to replace unhealthy 'props' with more constructive ones).

Think about the things you already do to unwind your mind and your body. You may be surprised by how many things there are – you probably instinctively try to manage your stress levels without even knowing you are doing it. At the end of a hectic day, perhaps you watch TV, listen to (or play) music, read a good book or go out with a friend. You might already know that you love a long, hot bath, a game of football, a walk in the woods, some yoga, a comfy armchair, a delicious meal, a cup of chamomile tea when you're feeling wound up. You know the stress busters that work for you: it's just a question of making sure you actually *use* them.

How to timetable your stress busters:

1 First, agree with yourself that this is *important* and not self-indulgent. This is actually a proven psychological tool known to reduce stress. You are therefore doing yourself

(and everyone who cares about you) a favour by taking stress busters seriously.

2 Now, write down what you have to do tomorrow.

3 Think about how you are going to fit in a stress buster – even something small. Can you have a hot bath before bed? Can you take a brief walk in the park after lunch? Can you find half an hour to bake a loaf of bread/sit in the garden/call a friend/work on your jigsaw?

Timetabling a stress buster can make the difference between it being an idea and a reality. This tackles the 'I can't possibly find time for that' syndrome. And this, in itself, is stress-reducing (you don't have to stress any more about not having time to de-stress!).

* * * * *

Stress really is horrid, but you can tackle it. Think of this as your own House of Rest – you are building it yourself, brick by brick. Once your construction project is underway you really will start to feel better. And when it is finished, you will be able to enjoy your life so much more. Try it and see.

NOTES FOR CARERS

'One may safely say, a nurse cannot be with the patient, open the door, eat her meals, take a message, all at one and the same time. Nevertheless the person in charge never seems to look the impossibility in the face.'

Florence Nightingale, *Notes on Nursing*, 1859

Caring for a loved one can be extremely stressful. That 'feeling overloaded' is often infectious – it can quickly affect an entire family, making life really difficult. Add to this any fears that stress itself might make a health problem worse, and you get a spiralling situation. To stop this – or turn things around, if it is happening already – try to:

1 **Educate yourself** Find out whether there is a (medically verified) relationship between stress and your loved one's health problem. The best way to do this is to talk to their medical team. The chances are you'll discover that it is not stress per se that causes health problems. Rather, it is the way we respond to stress that is bad for us (for example, finishing the bottle of wine, lighting a cigarette, or ignoring important dietary advice). It is no fun being stressed, but if you find sensible coping strategies then the stress itself is very unlikely to be harmful. What's more if you remove the worry and guilt associated with stress, you remove a whole layer of the stress itself.

2 **Help your loved one to understand their stress** It's important that they recognise how they tend to respond when stressed – this way they can do something about it. (The same goes for you, too!) You may also be able to take steps to avoid unhelpful stress responses (for example, removing alcohol/cigarettes/unhealthy snacks from the house).

3 **Arm yourself with stress-busting strategies** The coping strategies in this chapter are all 'evidence based'. This means one thing: they work! Use the strategies yourself, and see if you can encourage your loved one to use them too. Managing stress is very hard – so don't forget to reward yourself for your efforts.

4 **Seek (and accept) help** – either for yourself or your loved one. Stress comes down to overload – the sense that you can't meet the demands put on you. Getting help is a vital step to ending this feeling of overload.

❝Mum got really stressed after her accident. She was trying to do all that she had been doing before, plus her physiotherapy. I had to use time-management techniques I use at work to help her focus on what was important and let some things go. I did feel a bit harsh, and it wasn't easy at the time, but she now says it helped her to think straight.❞

Callum, 31, son of Annabel, 55,
who broke both legs in a car crash

FOUR

LOW SPIRITS

DEPRESSION AND WHAT TO DO ABOUT IT

'Nobody has suffered more from low spirits than I have done so I feel for you. 1) Live well and drink as much wine as you dare. 2) Go into the shower bath with a small quantity of water at a temperature low enough to give you a slight sensation of cold – 75 or 80 (degrees). 3) Amusing books. 4) Short views of human life not farther than dinner or tea. 5) Be as busy as you can. 6) See as much as you can of those friends who respect and like you 7) and of those acquaintances who amuse you. 8) Make no secret of low spirits to your friends but talk of them fully: they are always the worse for dignified concealment.'

Letter from Sidney Smith, writer and cleric, to Lady Georgiana Morpeth, 16 February 1820

Why am I depressed?

Depression and health problems go hand in hand. Fifteen to 25 per cent of people who have had a heart attack, for example, feel depressed a year or more later. Indeed, low mood is so common after a heart attack that it actually has its own name – 'homecoming depression' – and gets a mention in the learned *Manual of Cardiovascular Diagnosis and Therapy* by Joseph S. Alpert, et al. (2002).

It is a similar story for other illnesses, operations and accidents: 15–40 per cent of cancer survivors experience some form of depression in the first year after treatment. About 20 per cent of people who fracture a hip and have to have an emergency hip replacement are depressed several months later (they were not depressed before). One quarter of those who have a traumatic accident are depressed one year on. And up to a third of those who are involved in motor vehicle accidents (whether in the vehicle, on a bicycle or as a pedestrian) are depressed three months later. Many of these people are still depressed up to, and beyond, the first anniversary of the accident. Up to a third of people who suffer a stroke go on to develop depression. Low mood is also a very common side effect of surgery: for example, longer-term depression is found in up to 30 per cent of people who have undergone abdominal surgery. Indeed, depression after hysterectomy is so common that clinical researchers have suggested that it should be considered as one of the major post-operative complications.

You get the picture: if you are feeling low, or downright depressed, you are in very good company.

> ❝I don't know what to call it. Is it depression, frustration or just life? All I know is that I can't do half the things I used to do before the accident. My character has changed, I am irritable most of the time, sometimes I'm even weepy, which I never used to be. I don't enjoy things like I used to do, in fact I have stopped doing loads of things I used to do and when I think about the future I can't see it getting any better. ❞
> **Kevin, 58, broke his pelvis and leg in a car crash**

Understanding depression

There are many highly effective ways to tackle your mood and feel better – you don't have to 'live with it' – but before you get down to the nitty-gritty, it is very useful to understand how depression works. Depression:

- Can be triggered by something very stressful or difficult – and illness, surgery or accident certainly fit that bill.

- Can have biological causes (that is, a chemical imbalance in the brain).

- Can be induced by some medical interventions (for example, it is a known short-term side effect of anaesthesia, and is also associated with some forms of chemotherapy).

- Is not a sign of weakness or self-indulgence.

- Is not something that you can just 'snap out of'.

- Is not your fault.

- Is not a 'thing' that you 'have'. It is a cluster of 'symptoms' – in your feelings, your body, your behaviour or your thoughts – that together make you feel different, unhappy and stuck.

Diagnosis: how do you know if you're depressed?

Everyone feels down sometimes, but when does the blues become 'depression'? There is no scan or blood test to diagnose depression. Scientists have tried very hard to pinpoint a way to diagnose it reliably. After endless elaborate scientific research studies, and long, detailed, complex questionnaires, this is what they've come up with. One of the most effective ways to diagnose depression is simply to ask the person two questions:

1 During the past month, have you often been bothered by feeling down, depressed, or hopeless?

2 During the past month, have you often been bothered by little interest or pleasure in doing things?

If you answer yes to these two questions, then you may be depressed.

Am I depressed?

As a rough guide, if you find that you have at least five of the symptoms below, and they last a minimum of two weeks, then you may be showing signs of depression. But, frankly, if you are depressed, you probably already know it.

The symptoms of depression:

1 Feel sad most of the time

2 Cry often

3 Feel helpless, hopeless or worthless

4 Tired/lethargic/lacking in energy

5 Experiencing appetite changes

6 Having trouble sleeping (including waking in the night and early in the morning)

7 Feel you've lost your libido

8 Thinking negative things about yourself, the world and the future

9 Losing interest in people and withdrawing from others

10 Not enjoying activities that you used to enjoy

11 Thinking about harming yourself

12 Finding it hard to concentrate

13 Going over and over the same thoughts in your mind (getting stuck with certain thoughts)

14 Feeling slow, mentally

15 Not looking after yourself (for example paying less

attention to your appearance, personal hygiene, or using alcohol or drugs too much)

16 Doing less activity

If you recognise many of these depressed signs, but you didn't think you were depressed, then you have just put your finger on a major problem:

> How on earth can we distinguish the symptoms
> of depression from the straightforward
> consequences of being physically unwell?

Many of the physical symptoms on the list, such as appetite, sleep or energy level changes, are also perfectly normal in people who aren't in the least bit depressed, but have just had surgery, a heart attack, a stroke or any other major health issue.

It isn't helpful to get too hung up on a depression 'diagnosis' when you've been ill or had an injury. What matters is how you feel in yourself. If you feel low, then that is how you are.

Why now?

Health problems do not just disrupt your daily life. They change your long-standing plans and ambitions. They force you to face things you didn't want to face, maybe even to be someone you didn't want to be. This can make you feel very down.

You may be facing:

1 Loss:

⑥As the stroke was happening to me I could feel my body disintegrating. It was like watching one of those old factory towers collapse – you know, when they do a controlled explosion – only my stroke felt like a very uncontrolled explosion. But everything happened so fast after that I sort of forgot it and just got on with trying to stay alive. It is only now, months later, that I find myself thinking about that image. It makes me feel so desperately sad. That tower was me – tall, strong, powerful. And now I feel like a pile of rubble. 9

Maurice, 74, had a stroke

2 Facing a different future:

6 I was diagnosed with cancer while pregnant. I know I am incredibly lucky to have my little girl, and I do thank God for her. But I always imagined having a big family and, sometimes, just sometimes, I feel like I have lost the future that I planned, and I long for it. 9

Helene, 32, had breast cancer

3 Facing changes:

6 I felt incredibly depressed when the doctor told me I would never play football properly again. 9

Fergus, 26, had a skiing accident

4 Feeling vulnerable:

6 I have taken early retirement. It was a very difficult decision because I loved nursing, I always felt proud saying that I was a nurse. Also I am single and the effect on me financially was not ideal. But in the end I realised that I could not keep both my work and my health under control, so I had to choose my health. 9

Janelle, 57, had an aneurism

How to tackle your depression

There are many highly effective ways to tackle depression, in mind and body. This chapter is your toolkit.

Step one: get some exercise

This is your number-one depression-fighting strategy. If you only do one thing about your mood, make it this. Up-to-date scientific research shows that 30 minutes a day of regular exercise such as walking is just as good, if not better, than antidepressants for treating people with mild to moderate depression.

You may now have your head in your hands. Thirty minutes of exercise every day can seem like an impossible task, even for people who haven't had a major health issue. But when you are depressed it can seem out of the question. The good news is that it's just as effective to break it up into 10-minute slots, so you don't have to tackle the 30 minutes in one go.

Just do it

If trying to think about what kind of exercise you would like to do is completely impossible because you don't like anything any more (or you don't like anything you can do now), the answer is simple: just pick something. If you wait until you want to exercise, or can find the perfect activity, or are 'well enough' to do what you might like, you may be waiting for a very long time – even without depression it can be hard to get going. So, pick something that sounds doable, or better still, join someone you know who is already doing an activity. If you can hardly move your body now, let alone walk for 10 minutes, you may think this doesn't apply to you; however, there are always ways to exercise – even while sitting down! See Chapter 10 for ideas.

❝I got very depressed after my hysterectomy. I withdrew, couldn't bring myself to return to work. I'd made a good physical recovery but it was the emotional side that I struggled with. A friend who was going through a nasty divorce suggested we walk together, but I felt I was rotten company. She persisted and eventually I gave in. We got a copy of our local *AtoZ* and at the end of each walk we highlighted the roads we had covered. I controlled how far we went, and our speed, so I never felt any pressure. We did this for months. It became a challenge to highlight every road on every page – and we talked constantly. It was the best cure. We're both too busy to do it daily now, but we still walk every weekend, rain or shine.❞

Carolyn, 57, had a hysterectomy

For more detailed advice on exercise see Chapter 10.

Step two: use mindfulness techniques

Like physical exercise, mindfulness is a highly effective way to tackle depression. It teaches you new ways to approach, acknowledge and accept difficult or painful emotions. It allows you to break old habits and patterns of thinking and behaving – and to feel less 'stuck'. Some mindfulness exercises can seem a bit abstract, but studies show that they really do work, so have faith. In fact, reliable studies show that an eight-week mindfulness course (one 2–3 hour session a week, with up to an hour a day of home practice) is actually as effective as antidepressants in treating mild to moderate depression. Crucially, mindfulness is also a particularly effective way to reduce your risk of becoming depressed again later.

The mindfulness exercises in this book are really just tasters – it is a really good idea to go on a mindfulness course, if you possibly can (see Resources).

Try this: breathing space

This is a key mindfulness technique to use when you are feeing upset or troubled. When you notice yourself feeling this way, it's time for a three-minute breathing space. This is as easy as it sounds. When you notice yourself having difficult emotions, you simply take a moment to 'tune in' to what's going on with your emotions, thoughts and body.

1 Try to notice what's happening without being judgemental. You don't need to stop or change anything; for example, you might think to yourself: 'Low mood has hit', 'The self-critical thoughts are here', 'Motivation has vanished', 'I've tensed up.'

2 Once you've tuned into what's happening, try to focus on your breathing. There is no right or wrong way to breathe, just notice how your body feels as you breathe in and out, in and out. When your mind wanders – and it will – just go back to your breath and the sensations of air flowing in and out. Your breath is your anchor – keep coming back to it.

3 Now try to notice what's happening in the rest of your body. Pay particular attention to any parts that feel tight, uncomfortable or painful. As you breathe out, gently try to let go in those parts of your body. Then just let it be – just notice and accept any tightness, pain or discomfort.

Although this is called the three-minute breathing space don't get hung up on the time. It might take more or less than three minutes to feel calmer – just do what seems right. The only thing to bear in mind is that this isn't a long, time-consuming meditation. It is supposed to be a rapid response – your few moments of 'breathing space'.

Breathing space is a haven from the downward spiral of pain and distress. You'll need to practise and persevere with it, but it can offer you a different way of responding to difficult emotions. This simple technique really can help you break the bonds of your own depressed mindset.

Step three: tackle depressed thoughts

If you've read Chapter 2, you will now understand that how you feel is strongly influenced by your thoughts. (If you haven't, read pages 54–8, 'Your thoughts and why they matter', that's your starting point, then come back here.)

Your thoughts are not always helpful or realistic. It is very easy to fall into cunning little traps. Depression has its own very common Thought Traps. It is worth looking through these so that you will be alert when they crop up in your own head.

Common depressed Thought Traps

Depressed Thought Traps tend to be absolute and extreme. Life isn't black or white, but when depression hits it can seem very dark indeed. It is likely, as you start to pinpoint your low thoughts, that a few of these common Thought Traps will crop up:

- Labelling yourself: 'I'm pathetic', 'I'm weak.'

- Mental filtering: when this happens, it's as if you're wearing a pair of glasses that filter out what you're actually achieving. 'I can't clean as well as I once did' (you've filtered out the fact that you're cleaning the house in the first place).

- Unrealistic or harsh expectations: 'I ought to be better by now', 'I should be able to walk better than this', 'I must not let my feelings show.'

- Fortune-telling: 'Things will never be any good again', 'I'm never going to be able to support my family again.'

- All-or-nothing thinking: 'If I can't get back to full-time work I will be useless.'

- Catastrophising/thinking the worst: 'My life is over', 'I cannot recover.'

Having identified some of the ways in which your thoughts get trapped when you are depressed, it is time to look at and question them.

Your 'case for the defence'

What's the evidence? See if you can cross-examine your own thoughts. Ask yourself questions, such as: am I wearing 'filter glasses' that stop me from seeing things I'm actually achieving? Was my day completely blank, or have I actually achieved tasks today? How much effort have I had to put into getting through today? Am I labelling and blaming myself for everything that goes wrong? Do I think anything that goes right is a fluke or down to the kindness/support of others? Am I predicting the future and writing it or myself off? Do other people agree or disagree with my view of myself, the world and the future? If they disagree, what is their perspective?

What are the mitigating circumstances? Ask yourself whether you are expecting yourself to function as you did before your health problem. Are you filtering out the fact that you've been through the mill? You may be expecting yourself to 'bounce back' overnight, or you may be imagining that basic tasks (getting up, brushing your teeth, talking to others, concentrating on a newspaper article) should be as easy as they were before. If these things now take far more effort, try to give yourself credit for this effort. Ask yourself how reasonable your expectations are. See if you're using 'shoulds', 'musts', 'oughts' to drive yourself forward ('I *should* be better', 'I *must* not cry', 'I *ought* to be walking by now'). These ways of thinking can be overwhelming. It may be time to cut yourself some slack, be kind to yourself. This isn't about making excuses or lowering your standards. It's about recognising what you've been through.

Is thinking like this fair or helpful? Are these ways of thinking fair and does it help me to get going again or feel better?
Am I thinking in all-or-nothing/black-or-white/extreme ways?
Is this realistic – isn't life really more about shades of grey? Is
telling myself that I am a failure helping me to tackle my low
mood or making me feel more helpless? How have I got
through similar situations in the past? What helped me to
cope? Can I use these strategies now or are there other ideas I
can put into practice? What would I say to someone else in this
situation? (It's amazing how many of us have double standards:
one harsh rule for me and one realistic rule for everybody
else.) Ask yourself if you would say these things to a sister,
child, friend or colleague: 'You are pathetic', 'You are weak',
'You are nowhere near as skilled as you used to be', 'You'll
never get better.' No – you wouldn't dream of saying these
things, would you? That would be wholly unreasonable and
harsh. And yet, when depressed, we say things like that to ourselves without hesitation.

Building your case for the defence against depressed Thought
Traps is about opening yourself up to the idea that there might
be another way of looking at your situation. You don't have to
accept, without question, your first, automatic, harsh and
unhelpful thought.

❛I was so low for a long time after it happened. I kept
telling myself that I was lucky to be alive, and losing my
arm was a small price to pay for life. But deep down I also
thought that my old life was over and I wasn't sure that I
could face the new life ahead of me. I tried to pull myself
together. I told myself I should be coping better, staying
cool, calm and composed, not letting my feelings get the
better of me. But that just made me worse, more tense,
more wound up, more depressed. Talking to a

psychologist helped me realise that ignoring the loss and setting myself such high standards wasn't helping me or the people I love. She helped me to deal with my sadness, to cut myself a bit of slack, to take things slowly and to recognise what I was doing instead of what I could no longer manage. ❞

Richard, 47, had his arm amputated after an infection

Or, as good old Sidney Smith wrote 200 years ago in his letter to Lady Morpeth: 'Don't be too severe upon yourself or underrate yourself, but do yourself justice.'

TIP

The inquisition

You do not have to go hammer and tongs at your cross-examination. In fact, when you're feeling low, it's easy for your 'barrister' to get very harsh and aggressive. If you can, make your defence barrister incredibly kind, gentle and understanding. Make them non-judgemental, and compassionate (this isn't court-room realism, remember, it's only happening inside your head). The cross-examination should be more of a curious process of enquiry than a brutal drubbing.

Step four: tackle depressed behaviour

How you feel, emotionally, affects how you behave. When you are depressed, getting out of bed to face the day can feel like a Herculean task. But depressed behaviour (such as withdrawing from friends, or pulling the duvet over your head and not getting up at all, or the opposite – rushing around doing things with little enjoyment) tends to bolster, or even deepen, a depression. One key to tackling depressed behaviour is to find a balance: you want activity that is productive and manageable without being exhausting or overwhelming. This isn't easy, let alone intuitive. But there are several ways to make it happen.

Try this: write a daily plan

When you are low, you lose confidence and Thought Traps spring up at you telling you that you should be doing more/better/faster. If you plan out your day in advance you won't wake up and think, 'How am I going to get through today?' You won't feel you've 'achieved nothing' or are 'useless'. And you won't get into a muddle, thinking that there are things you should be doing but are failing to do. You are following your daily plan. You are simply doing what you're supposed to do, when you're supposed to do it. Life can't always be packaged up into controllable chunks, of course, but there are probably some 'core' activities that you do most days. So plan these into each day. Try to include time for:

- Personal hygiene – shower/bath/shave/cleaning teeth
- Eating/drinking
- Activity/exercise
- Employment or work around the home (DIY, shopping, cleaning)
- Social contact
- Interest or hobby

Tick off the tasks as you achieve them. This gives you solid evidence of what you are managing, even when your Thought Traps tell you that you've done 'nothing'. It does sound silly to plan to brush your teeth at 8.00 am, then tick it off a list. But try it – it is astonishing how helpful it can be, when you are feeling low, to feel you are achieving simple daily tasks, that you are more in control and that the day isn't just this messy, looming thing.

> ❝I found the idea of not waiting until you feel like doing something but doing it anyway very helpful: it got me motivated again. Crossing items off my daily schedule also helped me to feel like I was actually doing something. My life had felt very out of control, and it was a relief to feel that I had finally taken some control back.❞
> **Priyanka, 47, had breast cancer**

Do something enjoyable

A vital part of kicking depression is to do things you actually enjoy. Fun isn't a luxury; it is a vital strategy in overcoming low mood. The problem is, when you're feeling down, it can be genuinely hard to come up with anything you think you'd enjoy.

Try this: set a goal

1 **Think about the things you've enjoyed previously** It can be anything – work, leisure, family, spirituality, fitness, socialising, education or learning and hobbies.

2 **Find one thing that you are not doing** but that is fun. Make it important. Pick something you used to do, which you loved but have dropped since being ill, or find something new that you've always wanted to try. If neither of these seems doable, then come up with something new and enjoyable-sounding that you feel you could manage. Make doing this your goal.

3 **Can you achieve your goal today?** If so, that's great. But many goals take more time. You'll probably need a series of steps or shorter-term goals to get there.

4 **Look at your goal and work out the steps you need to get there** For example, if you want to get back to knitting baby clothes, the first step may be finding your old knitting needles, buying some new wool and ordering a pattern book. The next step may be practising your basic stitches, starting off with a scarf, before moving on to the ultimate goal of booties and bobble hats. The same goes for taking up golf again, or trying hang-gliding or digging the bestseller you are writing out of your bottom drawer. Think enjoyable baby steps, leading towards the ultimate goal.

TIP

Don't give up

At first, all this may not feel much 'fun' at all. But if you keep going with your goals, and with scheduling your day, you'll slowly realise that you are making progress. Gradually, you'll start to enjoy things, and look forward to them. Be patient – this can take a long time, but it will happen eventually if you are persistent.

SMART GOAL SETTING

Goals are pointless unless they're realistic. If they are unrealistic, you're only going to set yourself up for failure – and that's the last thing you need. Check that your goal is SMART:

1 Specific: don't just say, 'Go out more', say 'Go for a day at the beach.'

2 Measurable: how will you know if you've achieved what you set out to do? ('Did I get to the beach?')

3 Achievable: spending a whole day out of the house may be your ultimate goal, but start small – half an hour on the beach may be much more achievable at first. Remember, don't set yourself up for failure.

4 Relevant: only pick goals that are meaningful ('The beach is a place I love – I've had tons of happy times there and the kids love it.').

5 Timely: ask yourself, 'Is now really the right time to work on this goal?' (If it's November, then a day on the beach might be awful – maybe you could postpone that one until summer.)

Antidepressant medication

If you are very depressed and stuck, medication ('antidepressants') can kick-start a recovery process. There are, of course, pros and cons.

PROS	CONS
Antidepressants can work very well for many people (they usually take a couple of weeks to kick in)	They are not effective for everyone or every kind of depression
They are not addictive for most people	It may take a while to find the right antidepressant for you ('one Prozac does not fit all')
They have far fewer debilitating side effects than they once had	They can have side effects, such as loss of libido or weight changes
They may lift your mood enough for you to start trying other methods (such as exercise, social life, interests) to treat your own depression	You may have had it with tablets – if you feel like you're already rattling when you move because you take so many pills, it can be hard to take even more

Antidepressants are most effective when used in combination with a talking therapy, but NHS psychological services are very oversubscribed, so doctors may get their prescription pad out first when what you really need most is talking therapy (see below) – or talking therapy plus antidepressants.

Talking to a therapist

If your doctor prescribes antidepressants, it is always worth asking for talking therapy as well. A combination of the two will maximise your chances of a fast and strong recovery. It is always good to talk to family or friends about how you feel. They can (hopefully!) listen, offer advice and give a new perspective; however, unlike a trained therapist, your loved ones are always going to bring their own needs, issues and expectations to the table. This can become complex (for you and them), and sometimes may not be too helpful.

'I can't go on'

If you just want the suffering to stop, you don't want to wake up, or you think 'it's not worth carrying on', please don't think you are alone. People often feel weak or stupid or crazy when they have these thoughts, but if you are thinking these things, you're actually very brave – you are carrying on, despite these thoughts, and that takes courage. There is, however, a crucial difference between exhausted thoughts ('How much longer can I go on like this?', 'I wish this suffering would end') and active suicidal thoughts where you actually plan how you'll take your own life.

If you find yourself having thoughts about wanting to harm or kill yourself, and how you might do it, then you need to get professional help: **right now**. Go to your doctor immediately and tell them, honestly, how you are feeling. If it is out of hours, go to A&E and explain that you need help. If all this is too much, pick up the phone and call an emergency suicide-prevention helpline, such as The Samaritans (see Resources).

If you were in extreme physical pain you wouldn't stay at home trying to manage the horrible symptoms on your own, you'd get medical help – very fast. But somehow, for extreme emotional pain we seem to have a different standard. There is a notion that we should just pull ourselves together, or soldier on – that it is something we have to face alone (it isn't) and that time heals. Well, time may or may not heal, but if you are at a point where you are thinking about ending your life, then you do not have time. You need help right now. There are many people out there who want to, and can, help you: you can get through this.

Tackling loneliness

Loneliness or isolation can be a major problem in many people's lives, even without a health issue. But ill health or injury can certainly make the problem worse. Loneliness can actually hamper your recovery; it can make you less likely to get help, more likely to feel low, and therefore less likely to take good care of yourself: to eat well, to follow new regimes, to take pills on time, to do any rehabilitation exercises. In other words, if you are lonely, it is a good idea to do something about it.

Breaking out of loneliness can feel like an impossible task. But there are many ways to reach other people – even if you feel you are very limited by your health. Here are some ideas:

Be bold If you feel alone, the first thing to do is ask yourself whether you are really as isolated as you think. Perhaps you have a few phone numbers but assume that none of those people would want to hear from you. This could be your low mood talking. It is easy to 'mind-read' (assume people think something when you actually have no real evidence for that). Bravery might be called for – sometimes you have to be bold, and just pick up the phone, or send the email, or write the post-card. You may get some disappointing knock-backs. But equally, you may get in touch with someone who is happy to hear from you, and this could be a valuable first step towards breaking out of isolation.

Find a regular activity An adult education course, perhaps a writing class, or a specific support group, will give you regular contact with other people. They may not all be bosom buddies. But just having something in the diary, so that you are guaranteed to see people every few days, is a great start. A health charity for your particular health concern may run local groups where you can meet people who have been through similar experiences.

Be altruistic If you are up to it, you could turn the whole thing around and help others by volunteering. There is, in fact, firm scientific evidence to show that altruism – helping others – has a positive influence on low mood. Volunteering can be a great place to start (see Resources). The wise old Sidney Smith in 1820 knew this when he advised Lady Morpeth to 'do good and endeavour to please everybody of every degree'.

❝I took early retirement from nursing. I'd given 35 years of my life to others and I needed to prioritise myself for a change. Initially, though, I became quite depressed. I am single, most of my friends were linked to work and I became very isolated. My doctor was fantastic. She said she'd give me antidepressants in one month's time, but before then I should take up some voluntary activity. I joined the local stroke support group, found a yoga class and volunteered with Age UK. I didn't go back for the antidepressants.❞

Angela, 57, had a stroke

Go online If your physical health (or mood) make it particularly difficult to get out of the house, social networking on the Internet is worth considering, even if you're not the Facebook generation. Communication has changed a lot. You can now Skype someone halfway across the world or instant message them for a virtual chat. You could consider signing up to Facebook, or writing a blog or joining an online chat room. It is actually possible to form deeply supportive (as well as light and frivolous) relationships with people you've never physically met. If you are feeling unconfident or shy, these 'once removed' relationships can be invaluable.

❝One of the best things that happened to me when I was recovering from my car crash was that my son introduced me to Facebook. I was so depressed after being in hospital, then in plaster, and still in pain. I began to follow what was happening to many of the people whom I love, especially my children, grandchildren, nephews and nieces. I loved seeing their new photos going up, and hearing their news, and it made me feel connected to them without being a burden. When I was on Facebook I was also thinking about others, not myself, and that was such a relief!

Sandra, 66, injured in a car crash

Give yourself time to heal

In the 'old days' people recognised that a patient had to recover not just from the physical trauma but from the emotional trauma too – the shock and fear of illness or injury. Dr John Bryant in his 1927 book, *Convalescence*, called this a 'disorganisation of the nervous system, both mental and motor'. Clearly, it would be silly to hanker nostalgically after the medicine of days gone by. Taking the air, after all, went hand in hand with leeches and bloodletting and mercury baths. Modern medicine is fantastic, but it is not magic. Today's hi-tech treatments can still be traumatic. They can have a powerful, often destructive and long-term effect on mood. The problem is that, nowadays, few people recognise that it can take a long time to heal, emotionally.

Try this: writing to heal

James Pennebaker, a professor of psychology in Texas, has spent his career looking at how writing about upheavals in life can improve physical and mental health. He recommends setting aside 20 minutes a day for four days in a row to write about your deepest emotions and thoughts in relation to difficult experiences in your life.

1 Write continuously for those 20 minutes, not worrying about the spelling, structure or any other 'literary' thing. It is private.

2 Get rid of the writing once it's done (or at the end of the four days): press the delete button, tear up the paper. This is 'writing to heal', not to share, let alone publish.

3 It is common to feel a bit down after your 20 minutes of writing – it is one of those 'you'll feel worse before you feel better' situations – but if you become very distressed, change what you are writing about – or stop.

4 Do not do this for more than four days in a row – enough is enough!

Reward yourself

You probably aren't going to like this section much. Most of us don't like to boast about our achievements, even to ourselves. And when we're feeling down, we're even less likely to pat ourselves on the back. But, in fact, rewarding yourself, and showing yourself some compassion and kindness is *vital*. It's a bit like dog training: the pooch is going to sit much quicker if you're doling out tasty doggy treats.

Rewards and compassion help us to build our confidence and motivation, but perhaps even more importantly they (think about that pooch) reinforce our learning. If something has a happy, positive consequence, we'll do it again, and again, and again. (See page 138 for more on compassion – and why it matters *a lot*.)

Try this: use your words

Think about how you reacted when someone you love achieved something brilliant – your child getting good marks in an exam, your partner getting a great job. What did you say to them? Think about this briefly before looking at the next paragraph.

You probably said something like: 'That's fantastic, you

worked really hard for that. I am really proud of you. Well done.' Perhaps you added a tangible reward – a congratulations card, a gift for the clever child, a photo to mark the occasion. You might even have gone on to talk about what the next step might be.

When it comes to your own achievements, particularly when you are feeling low, this doesn't happen. Thought Traps kick in: labelling, harsh expectations, filter glasses. We say cruel and unreasonable things to ourselves ('Yes, I swam a length, but I used to swim twenty!'). When you are low you need to work on being kinder to yourself. You've somehow got to replace the harsh, critical commentary with a realistic, balanced picture of what you've achieved.

It can help to have a few phrases (jotted down if you just can't remember them at the time) that you can – and will – say to yourself when you achieve something.

Encouraging words:

- 'I am trying my best.'
- 'That took a lot of effort.'
- 'I am managing a bit more each day.'
- 'This is a setback – I have had one before, I know what to do.'
- 'I did really well.'
- 'That was impressive given how low I am today.'

More tangible rewards

It's good to give yourself more tangible rewards too. These don't have to be wildly expensive gifts – a small bunch of flowers or a new magazine can very effectively mark the fact that you've done something. Rewards can also be experiential – a visit to a garden, a phone call to a good friend. So, plan out some rewards in advance – it can be hard to think of a treat on the spur of the moment. If you have made yourself a short list of possible treats, you'll cut out the stressful thinking process. Then you only have to consider which reward to choose this time.

Really?

Yes, really. Rewarding yourself is not silly nonsense that you can skip. The psychological value of rewards is backed up by a lot of solid scientific research. Numerous research studies show that rewarding your achievements, however small, will help to tackle your low mood.

Soothing yourself

In 1844 a French doctor, Dr Vidard-Dupin, wrote that the job of a 'Convalescent Physician' was to 'produce in the patient a tranquil spirit', to 'see that he avoided all excesses' and 'to allow him, whenever possible, any especially desired foods'. Modern research confirms that 'self-soothing' is a vital psychological technique for anyone recovering from illness or injury. Soothing yourself (sadly, no one else is likely do it for you these days) can boost your mood. It is a highly effective tool in combating depression.

When you were an overwrought baby you were rocked, stroked and cradled. The adults around you responded to you compassionately. Soothing comes in different forms – what soothes one person may enrage another. Only you will know what soothes you. Usually, though, soothing comes from engaging the senses: taking a bubble bath, being given a big hug, buying a bunch of sweet-smelling flowers, listening to music, having a massage, making a nice cup of tea, taking a stroll in the sun – all of these (and many more) can be highly effective 'soothers'. Try to work out what soothes you. Make a (long) list. Use that list when you are feeling like all the goal-setting and planning and rewarding is just too much.

Try this: a soothing visualisation

Visualisation is a relaxation technique where you take yourself to a calm place in your mind. Here's how:

1 Sit or lie somewhere quiet, comfortable and warm, where you won't be disturbed. Give yourself between 5 and 15 minutes for this – or longer.

2 Picture an imaginary place that works for you. You have to be realistic here. If you hate being alone, then a desert island isn't actually going to be that relaxing. You'd be better off imagining yourself on a busy beach on the Costa del Sol. To work out a good place, try to think about what your body does when it's tense: do you feel hot, fidgety, buzzing – or do you slow down? If you get hot when tense, a sun-drenched desert island isn't a good idea. You might be better off in a cool wood, or on a breezy beach. Whether it's a room in your childhood home, an alpine mountaintop, a meandering river, a desert island or a busy park, the key is to keep your place meaningful for you. It doesn't have to be a real place, by the way – you're free to take yourself to the tropical paradise you've always longed to visit.

3 Picture your place as clearly as you can. Some people like to start by walking themselves down some steps in their mind's eye to a door. They open the door and step into their special place. Where are you? What can you see?

4 Now use all your senses: imagine the sounds, smells, tastes, feel of your place. Try to visualise what is soothing for you.

5 Let yourself spend time in this place that you have visualised. You may want to be still or you may want to move around. You may be in an observer's role, watching what is going on, or taking a more active role and getting involved in your imagery – having a swim, a dance, a stroll – whatever it is that works for you.

6 Bring your visualisation to a close: if you walked down some steps at the start, close the door behind you and walk back up them to end. Maybe you have a different path that you want to retrace. The important thing is to remind yourself that you can bring yourself back to this place any time you want to. This is your soothing skill.

* * * * *

Depression and low mood are, then, a big – if unfortunate – part of recovery. You are not odd or weak or self-indulgent if you feel low. You have been through a huge upheaval. It is fair enough, on all levels, to feel down, but this does not have to be 'it' from now on. Your mood can – and will – improve.

> ❛I spent the first year and a half crying. I thought my life was over. My speaking life as I knew it was over. I felt unbearably sad. But gradually I realised that the sadness comes and goes. I slowly realised I still like being around people, listening to them and trying to contribute in my own way. I go to the Stroke Association club in my area, I like to look good, so I choose my clothes carefully and put on my makeup. I have found an inner peace. I notice and appreciate the little things in life now – before I was always too busy.❜
>
> **Theresa, 57, had a stroke**

It takes courage and determination to cope with depression, but the strategies you have read about in this chapter are scientifically tried and tested – they have worked for hundreds of thousands of people, and they can work for you. Theresa has developed strategies of her own – she is getting out, focusing on things she enjoys, rewarding herself. She has severe mobility and speech problems, she can't do many of the things she used to, but after a long, dark period, she has found ways to feel better. And so can you. You may find that the strategies in this chapter don't come easy. You need to think a lot about them, you will need to be determined, and you may need help and support. Sometimes this can feel like another huge task. But it will pay off. There is no need to feel low or depressed in the long term, so start to tackle your mood today – even the smallest step is a great beginning. Keep going, and you will see results. This will get better.

NOTES FOR CARERS

> *'I think it is a very common error among the well to think that "with a little more self control" the sick might, if they chose dismiss "painful thoughts" ... This state of nerves is most frequently to be relieved by care in affording them a pleasant view, a judicious variety as to flowers, and pretty things.'*

Florence Nightingale, *Notes on Nursing,* **1859**

Looking after someone with depression can be incredibly ... well, depressing. It can be tiring, frustrating, demoralising and draining. It can be hard to understand why, when they've 'come through' a serious illness or injury, they can't just pick themselves up and get on with it. The desire to shake your loved one out of their 'painful thoughts' can be overwhelming. But Florence Nightingale was right: depression has nothing to do with self-control. Recovering from depression can be a long and hard process. What you need are ways to stay focused and sane under trying circumstances:

1 **Look after yourself** This is essential for any carer, but when you are looking after a depressed person it becomes completely vital. Someone else's unhappy view of the world can be very powerful, and it is easy for you to start feeling the same way. One simple 'protective' strategy is to find something you love doing – and do more of it. Whether it's

cross-country running, oil painting or seeing your friends, make sure you do 'your thing' regularly. This is not selfish or spoilt. It is a vital survival skill. And it will enable you to be a far better carer than if you are dragged down into a low mood yourself.

2 **Listen and talk** but don't try to be a therapist. It is very easy to get into a repetitive depressed conversational loop where you talk about the same grim thing over and over and get nowhere. To guard against this, try to set a time limit (say half an hour at a time) on discussions about their unhappiness. You cannot expect to talk someone out of their depression. All you can do is be there for them. Try not to dismiss what they say as silly or wrong, or say things like 'cheer up' or 'it could be worse'. Instead, try to use active listening skills where you give them your full attention, summarise or repeat back to them what they've said (so you're both sure you understand their point) and ask open questions (ones that can't simply be answered with a yes or no). This can help you to feel less helpless and your loved one to feel understood.

3 **Encourage them to *do* things** Depression crushes motivation, but if your loved one can see that they are in fact achieving things (even if they are small things, and the person does not value them at the time), this can gradually improve their mood. Physical activity and exercise are particularly effective ways to fight depression. Having said this, it can be extremely hard to get a depressed person to do anything. If you can't seem to get through to them, don't be hard on yourself. This is not your fault. If you can bear it, just keep trying.

4 **Encourage them to make time for rewards and soothing** (see pages 122–3). But don't do this for them – this has to be something that comes from them. If they reward their own efforts, they are likely to keep trying. Remember that you

need to do this for yourself too – you are making a huge
effort here and need encouragement as much as they do.

5 **Get help** If your loved one shows signs of wanting to harm
   him or herself, or talks about suicide, then get professional
   help quickly (start with your doctor). This is not a burden
   that you should carry alone. If you are concerned that they
   may act on these thoughts, take action immediately – take
   them straight to the doctor (without an appointment if
   necessary), or to A&E outside doctors' practice hours.

❝Liam was really depressed after his accident. He felt so
helpless back home with Mum and Dad. I wanted to take
all his pain away, like when he was a baby, but I couldn't. I
had to let him do things for himself. I was always
thinking up little things that he could do for me like
unloading the top shelf of the dishwasher – he couldn't
bend down to the lower shelf – or taking the bin to the
compost heap, helping me sort my finances – anything to
show him that he was useful. He did see a psychologist at
the burns unit and he is miles better now, but it was a
long and painful process for us all.❞

**Kate, 47, mother of Liam, 23, who suffered burns in
a kitchen accident**

FIVE

THE TRANQUIL SPIRIT

REBUILDING YOUR CONFIDENCE

'Various forms of mental disturbance may follow operation; genuine insanity may occur, but it is relatively rare.'

Le Roi Goddard Crandon and Albert Ehrenfried,
***Surgical After Treatment*, 1912**

Health troubles – no matter what they are – can shake your foundations. One of the biggest challenges to feeling better is working out how to feel strong and capable again, dealing confidently with whatever you have to face, both now and in the future. When your confidence is shaken, this can be quite a journey. Think of this chapter as your roadmap to the confident new you.

What is self-confidence?

Your self-confidence is an ever-changing mosaic, formed from the underlying beliefs that you have about yourself. You may or may not even be aware of some of these beliefs, but at any given moment you are making judgements on yourself ('I'm a good person', 'a demanding person', 'a loveable person', 'an unlovable person', 'a disorganised person', 'a friendly person' – or many of the above). You have a sense of how you handle certain situations; of your abilities and skills ('I can handle a difficult meeting', 'I get nervous speaking in public', 'I don't find it easy to meet new people', and so on). You also have ideas about how you look and function physically ('I am elegant', 'I am fat', 'My wrinkles are showing', 'I limp and look off-balance', 'I look normal').

All of these judgements, ideas and beliefs have roots in the past: the messages you received as a child, how you behaved as you grew up, your circumstances, the support you received, how you coped. But they are also influenced by the present. You are constantly monitoring how you are coping right now ('I am getting on well with these people', 'I am not making myself clear', 'I know what to do', 'I don't know what to do', 'I can't cope', 'I'm going to get through this', and so on). This running commentary is sometimes helpful and sometimes not, but it is not set in stone. In fact, it can be thrown into total disarray by a health crisis.

> ❝Before my heart attack I'd been training for a half marathon, I didn't smoke or drink much and I was losing weight. I thought of myself as relatively young, fit and healthy. All of that changed at 9.15 pm on the 16th of April when I had my heart attack. I totally lost confidence in my body and myself. I felt like I'd turned into an old man overnight. It affected my home life, my work, my happiness – everything.❞
>
> **Rasoul, 48, had a heart attack**

The reasons why ill-health can knock your confidence

Loss of your 'old self'

> ❝After treatment finished I expected to feel relief, but in fact I felt a sort of grief. I had lost the old happy-go-lucky

me and replaced her with this fearful, lost person. My
confidence in my body and in myself was really
shaken. 9

Sally, 43, had breast cancer

Changed roles If you have always been the driver, it can be
hard to sit in the passenger seat. If you were always the breadwinner, it can be hard not to get up and go to work. If you were
the one who looked after others, it can be hard to be looked after.

6 I have always had to provide for myself and I have
never taken a handout. Having to go on benefits has been
terrible. I have worked for 40 years and paid all my taxes
but I still feel like I am getting something for nothing.
This just isn't me. 9

Geraldine, 61, had necrotising fasciitis

Loss of trust in your body You felt you knew and understood
your body, but now you don't. You can't trust it. You don't quite
know what it might do next. This can be worrying and stressful.

6 It broke my heart to lose my driving licence after I had
my stroke. I worked as a mechanic and my hobby was
rebuilding classic cars and motorbikes. My life was
vehicles. When the DVLA took my licence I felt empty. I
didn't know who I was anymore. I wasn't sure there was
any point in trying to get better. 9

Colin, 72, had a stroke

Loss of confidence can be triggered by a single event. Colin's
entire self-image was challenged by one devastating result of
his stroke. His loss of 'ability' changed how he saw himself. His
self-confidence plummeted.

An erosion of self-confidence doesn't have to be sudden. It is often a drip-drip process; for example, your home environment may be booby-trapped with reminders of what you used to be able to do but now find hard (or can't do). The dog is by the door – 'I should take him for a walk.' The dishes are on the side, 'I must do the washing up.' The laptop is on the desk, 'I should check my emails.' Your exhausted partner is cooking another meal, 'I should be helping.' When you feel you are not managing to do things, you start to make judgements about yourself as 'failing' or 'weak' or 'helpless' or 'exhausted'. Your internal commentary follows suit ('I'm stuck, I'll always be like this', 'my life is ruined'). Before you know it, your mosaic of self-confidence is scattered all over the place.

TIP

It's not just about you

Often our confidence is knocked by other people. Unhelpful comments such as 'Wow, you are still using a stick!' or 'Not back at work yet?' or 'Surely you could be driving by now?' can make you feel that you are failing.

People generally mean well when they say these things. They really want you to 'get back to normal'. But their motivation is actually complicated. They want this for you, but they also want it for themselves. If you get better, then the world hasn't changed. This was just a blip, not an earthquake – it's not that unsettling. If something similar happened to them, they'd probably get better too. So, when people say these things, try to remind yourself that it's not just about you – there are other things going on here. Their comments are also about them dealing with an uncertain and scary world.

Losing self-confidence: the downward spiral

- You begin to realise that some of the physical changes are long term.
- You look at the roles and responsibilities that used to be yours, but aren't now, and you can't help thinking about how you used to be.
- Your thoughts grow negative: 'I used to be able to do so much more', 'I should be doing so much better.'
- You start to judge yourself harshly: 'I can't cook/clean/work/exercise like I used to' becomes 'I am no good at cooking/cleaning/working/exercising'.
- You start to avoid things you feel unconfident about: 'I can't play football like I used to. I can't play in my weekend team, so what's the point of kicking a ball around at home?' (Before you know it, the ball hasn't been touched for weeks or months.)

> ❝My friend told me about her neighbour who had thrown her stick away two weeks after her knee replacement. I was still hobbling around on a stick five months on. I felt like a huge failure.❞
>
> **Marlene, 75, had a knee replacement**

How to rebuild your confidence

The good news is that the pieces of your confidence can be picked up and rebuilt – and when you've done this you may well end up feeling stronger than ever before. It is actually not that complicated. There are two key elements to building up your confidence.

1 Doing things: achieving tasks, setting goals and reaching them (even if it took a long time and some very small steps)

   and

2 Recognising what you have done.

You probably know at least one gorgeous, super-clever person who manages to achieve much more than most people – but they feel they're just not good enough. They think that others are better than them. However much they achieve – an Olympic gold medal, an Oscar – nothing would make them feel confident. This is because they cannot recognise their role in reaching their goals.

These days, you might be focusing on what you can't do any more, rather than on what you can do. The first step towards a confident new you is to get to know (and like and admire) this person you have become. And to do that, you first have to acknowledge what you have lost.

COMMON LOSSES

- Trust in your body
- Time (with a young family perhaps, or from your retirement, or work life, or the holiday of a lifetime)
- Body parts
- A sense of security
- Bodily functions
- Your looks
- Money
- Roles or your job
- Your sense of who you are

Any of these losses can have a profound effect on your confidence and it is important to allow yourself to feel sad about them.

Try this: time to grieve

You are going to give yourself permission to feel sad about what you've lost. This isn't self-indulgent – it is a necessary part of feeling better.

1 Set yourself 'time to grieve': set a timer for 15 minutes, two to three times a week for no longer than four weeks. During this time, you are really going to indulge your grief – let rip. Let yourself think about all the things that have changed – you can look at old photos or films of yourself, write a journal or some poetry, draw a picture, listen to music – do anything at all that helps you to think about what you have lost.

2 Stop. When your time is up, move on – put away all your memory aids, do something constructive and enjoyable (watch a favourite movie, go out for a walk, eat dinner with a friend, and so on). Time to grieve is over for today.

It can be scary to give yourself permission to grieve. You might worry that you're taking the lid off a can of worms, but you are not. The 'worms' (the sadness) are there however busy you keep yourself, however many distractions you have. Time to grieve is a way to control the sadness: now you are taking control over when and how you face your loss. This is far better than waiting for the sadness to jump out at you when you least expect it.

Meet the new you

You may feel that you don't recognise yourself any more. You've lost 'everything'. The next step in rebuilding your confidence is to locate the parts of yourself that are still going strong. They might even have grown stronger because of what's happened to you.

Try this: 'behind the headlines'

This will help you to understand more about how you see yourself now, to accept the changes and losses, and to work out a way to live in this 'new normal'.

Try to find 10 to 15 minutes somewhere quiet, where you won't be interrupted. Get a pen and paper and jot down the answers to the following questions:

1 What was I like before this happened? How would you have described yourself before your health crisis ('I'm creative and arty'; 'I'm strong and independent', 'I'm the family provider', 'I'm the office clown', 'I'm a leader').

2 Now dig deeper. Yes, these are the 'headlines', but what's behind them? The hidden you: maybe you provided for your family or kept your colleagues in stitches, but who else are you? Ask yourself:

- What else did I do? The non-headline news stuff; for example, were you the person who could defuse a tense situation? Were you practical – could you fix fuses or bake a fancy birthday cake? Were you altruistic – helping the neighbours, thinking of others? Now ask:

- Has all that really changed? Some of the headlines might have been wiped out. Perhaps you aren't the provider or the office clown any more, but the quieter parts of who you are may well be going strong. In fact, these less showy, obvious roles are often far more important than any of the 'headlines'. They actually matter more than your pay packet, your spotless home or your 'salesperson of the year' badge.

3 Keep what you've written down and use it almost like a journal – go back to it, and maybe add things as they occur to you.

Or, try this: stand outside yourself

This is another way to delve behind the headlines. It's not easy to do this (modesty tends to kick in, or embarrassment, or lack of confidence), but ask yourself:

- What do people who love me see in me?
- Why do they like me?
- Why do they love me?
- What do I do for, or with, them?
- What would they say about my strengths and good qualities?

Or, try this: 'What am I not?'

It's a bit left field, but looking at yourself in this way really can give you a clearer perspective on who you are deep down. So now ask yourself: 'What am I not?'

Think of qualities you dislike in other people – selfishness, cruelty, rudeness, aggression, indecisiveness, over-indulgence – whatever is meaningful for you.

Write down:

'I am not [fill in the characteristic], because ...'

For example: 'I am not rude, because I always try to treat people politely and with respect', 'I am not demanding, because I try to compromise and I think about the needs of others as well as myself.'

'A recent example of this is [fill in the example].'

For example: ' I was polite to the cold-caller who just tried to sell me health insurance', or 'I told the nurse who was giving me a bed bath to look after the lady in the bed next to me who was distressed.'

Looking at yourself from all these different perspectives, and writing down your answers, puts you in touch with who you are, deep down. You can rebuild your confidence by recognising your inner strengths, qualities, skills and achievements. Doing this will help you to try new things. You will also feel a lot better about yourself.

How to be compassionate – *towards yourself*

Paul Gilbert, the psychologist who wrote about the gazelle's anxiety volume switch, also describes how we have evolved to soothe ourselves.

When you were a baby, and you were distressed, adults would soothe, reassure and calm you. They would hold you close and stroke you, and tell you that you were safe and secure. This is how human beings learn compassion. Eventually, this exposure to compassion allows us to develop our own ways to soothe ourselves once a 'threat' has passed. And in doing so, we automatically 'turn down the volume' on our distress. There is only one problem: difficult emotions such as anxiety, stress, anger or depression can interfere with our ability to be compassionate *towards ourselves*. We might still be compassionate to other people, but when it comes to our own distress, that volume switch is harder to find.

The good news is that if you're aware of this, you can do something about it: you can get your 'self-compassion muscles' working again so that you can soothe yourself, and thereby turn down the distress volume very effectively. Doing this will make a huge difference to your ability to feel better when upset, distressed, down, worried or angry. There are many ways to strengthen those 'self-compassion muscles'. All the strategies in this book are, in essence, designed to rebuild your soothing and self-comforting abilities – but some are especially important.

Learning to soothe yourself and reward yourself (page 121) are particularly vital strategies.

- Soothing yourself might be as simple as taking a hot bath or making yourself a warm drink when you are wound up, or saying to yourself, 'I am OK' or 'I will get through this', when you're worried or overwhelmed.

- Giving yourself rewards (either concrete, or just by thinking positive, bolstering things) helps to embed the changes you are trying to make so that they stick. It also helps you to realise that you played a part in all this – it was *you* who made the changes happen. You are effective. In fact, you are far more powerful than you might have thought.

In other words, although learning to be compassionate towards yourself might sound a bit woolly, it is actually a highly effective psychological tool – vital to the whole process of feeling better.

Try this: The Voice

Think of a voice that is warm, loving and very compassionate. It can be your own voice – perhaps the one you use with your own children when they're upset, or with other people you love. Or, it can be another person's loving and kind voice – either an imagined 'ideal' person or someone you actually know who fits that bill. This is The Voice.

The next time you are upset – worried, stressed, frightened, angry or depressed – you're going to try to summon up The Voice in your mind. The Voice does not try to change anything or get you to do anything – it is simply warmly and generously kind, loving and reassuring. It recognises your distress and it doesn't judge you. It understands. It soothes and comforts you. Now, try to actually hear the voice in your head saying comforting things (such as 'Poor you', 'You will get through this', 'You're doing your best', 'Keep going, you're doing really well' – or anything at all that you find comforting).

This exercise might feel strange and uncomfortable to begin

with, but remember, The Voice is in there, somewhere – it has been evolutionarily hard-wired inside you by your earliest experiences. It's just a question of finding it again. When you find The Voice, keep using it as often as you can. In time, The Voice will become your personal, compassionate 'volume control'.

Tackling avoidance

> ❝I'm not a sporty person but I used to use my exercise bike every day without fail. Since my surgery I just don't know if it would help, or make me worse. Plus, I know that it would be impossible for me to cycle 20k like I used to. I have got my husband to move the bike up into the loft so I don't see it each day.❞
> **Elaine, 52, had back surgery after falling down stairs**

When faced with something that scares us, the human instinct is avoidance: run, hide, don't look it in the eye. This is a hard-wired evolutionary response. If the sabre-toothed tiger is bearing down on you, then hiding in your cave is a great idea; however, for less physical threats, the instinct to avoid isn't helpful. When you avoid things that scare you they don't vanish, they fester. Over time this will eat away at your self-confidence.

Try this: look it in the eye

You may know exactly what it is you're trying to avoid (the mirror/your old friends/the route to the hospital/sex). Or it might be far less clear.

See if you can make a list of things you're avoiding. Be honest. Think about particular situations, places, activities or people that you are avoiding now. Of course, you may be avoiding some things that you used to do because they are physically impossible for you now, or because you have simply lost interest in them. If you could do something, but it no longer seems relevant or important to you, then this isn't really avoidance: your priorities have changed. And if you want to do it, but can't for some really concrete reason, this isn't avoidance; for example, Colin, who lost his driving licence, can't get back to driving – he's not avoiding it, it has been taken from him. However, if you care about it, and could do it but are worrying that you can't, then this is avoidance; for example, Elaine might not really need to hide that exercise bike in the attic.

Once you've worked out what it is that you're avoiding, you need to:

- Establish your 'goal': what exactly do you need to face/get back to/try?

- Build yourself a 'ladder'. Think about the steps you will need to take to get to that goal. The key here is to make the steps very small and manageable. Think about what is realistic for you, right now. You have to build up very gradually towards your goal. It could take weeks or longer to get there. Elaine, for example, wanted to get back to cycling for half an hour on her exercise bike. She asked her physio to help her establish a good starting point – the speed and distance to try at first. If she'd tried to leap back on and cycle at a mad pace for half an hour, she would have battered her confidence into the dust and never touched the bike again. But 5 minutes of gentle cycling was doable for her. After doing this every day for a week, she increased to 7 minutes. The next week she increased her speed. Then she increased her time the following week to 10 minutes. It took her two months, but she got there – and she is now cycling half an hour at a good speed every day. You may never get to where you once were, but your confidence will grow as you achieve the small steps you set yourself. The hare might leap ahead, but then he'll crash spectacularly. The steady old tortoise will get there.

TIP

Think through the practicalities

If you physically can't do something because you don't have the equipment, or other practicalities aren't in place, then it won't happen; for example, if you can't get to the pub because you can no longer drive, then your goal of socialising again will be scuppered before you even start. You therefore need to sort out a lift. Or a bus route. Or a bike. Or a taxi. Think logistics. Think equipment. Think practicalities. When Elaine realised she was avoiding her exercise bike, she decided to tackle it. But to do this she had to get her husband to take the bike back down to the kitchen. This sounds blindingly obvious, but the best intentions can be sabotaged by lack of 'equipment' or logistical hitches.

Do things!

When you lose confidence in yourself it is easy to stop doing things in general. Sometimes the path of least resistance is simply to let other people do things for you. But this can lead to a very restricted life. This is an extension of avoidance. There certainly may be many important things that you can't do at the moment (jogging/going to work/getting upstairs) but there will also be things you can manage (rehabilitation exercises/supporting a work colleague over the phone/taking a distance-learning course). Your goals don't have to be major physical activities. The more subtle, less physical achievements are no less important to rebuilding your confidence. The trick is to recognise the effort it takes you to do these things. Helping a grumpy teenager with their homework might, for example, involve as much effort as scoring the winning goal in your local five-a-side league match. The only difference is that the effort is intellectual and emotional rather than physical.

Recognise the things you do

When you were fit, young, healthy and busy, you probably achieved all sorts of physical, mental and emotional tasks every day without noticing them. But when your confidence has been knocked, it is vital to start recognising and valuing what you manage to do each day – even the smallest things.

If you set yourself a goal at the start of the day and you have achieved it by the end of the day, be sure to point this out to yourself: tick it off your list, write it down in an achievements notebook or tell your partner. These are the building blocks of confidence.

If you didn't manage your goal, look instead at how you handled the disappointment. Goal setting can be hit and miss. Did you crumble and collapse? Or have you kept going? Did you rethink your goal? Have you tried something else? Did you get support? Recognising how you cope when things don't go your way is an important part of rebuilding your confidence. Try to give yourself credit for coping. And if you didn't cope – you crumbled and collapsed – then give yourself a break: you probably needed to stop. You can always start again tomorrow.

Reward yourself

Tangible rewards remind you that you are, indeed, achieving things. They encourage you to keep going. Start with recognising what you've done *every* time you do it, no matter how small it seems. Words can be rewards. When you achieve something – even something small – try to say something to yourself like 'I did it!', or 'Hooray. I got there!' When you make more progress – a next step, a mini-milestone – you can add in more concrete rewards – a trip to the cinema, that fine shirt you've had your eye on, a bubble bath, a bar of chocolate.

This isn't daft. Reliable psychological studies show that rewards are absolutely KEY to changing our behaviour. So remember this: step, reward, step, reward.

Beware the 'Yes ... buts'

This is a common pattern when confidence is low: 'Yes, I made a lasagne, but I used to do it from scratch for 15 people without breaking a sweat.' We all do this to a certain extent, but confident people tend to bat these thoughts away automatically – the thought is a momentary lapse, not reality. But when your self-confidence is low you are more likely to fall into such Thought Traps, and stay in them. You will genuinely believe the thoughts. They will feel like reality.

Other common low-confidence Thought Traps include:

- Mind-reading: 'No one wants me here', 'They're staring at my scars', 'I'm letting my family down.'

- Self-blame: 'If I was a more upbeat person, I'd be over this by now', 'I'm ruining her life.'

- Harsh expectations: 'I shouldn't ever cry', 'I should be happy that I can move at all, even if it hurts', 'I mustn't feel sorry for myself.'

As ever, when you spot a Thought Trap it's time for your 'case for the defence'.

Build your 'case for the defence'

Example: Thought Trap – self-blame: 'I'm ruining her life.'

What's the evidence? Are you really ruining her life? Has she said so (and if she did, was it an angry outburst that she didn't really mean)? Is her life ruined, or is she in fact leading a life quite similar to the one before you were ill? Doesn't she actually love you? Think about what you do still offer: your love, support, sense of humour, kindness. Wouldn't she far rather live with you like this than not have you here at all?

What are the 'mitigating circumstances'? You've been through something extremely difficult. You have coped with enormous challenges and are continuing to cope, and so has your partner. Illness and injury change roles and relationships, it will take time for you both to get used to the new situation.

Is thinking like this fair or helpful? It is fair enough to acknowledge what has been lost and changed – you both have a lot to adjust to. But does thinking that you are 'ruining her life' help you in this process of adjustment? Does it help you to talk together about your concerns? Does it help you to try to rebuild your relationship or your confidence? Or does it in fact do the opposite – making you feel worse about yourself and less likely to find ways to improve the situation? Can you imagine saying, 'You're ruining your wife's life!' to your best friend or brother, if they were in a similar situation to you? Of course not – you know that would be harsh, untrue and unfair. So why say it to yourself?

Your body image

Body image and self-confidence go hand in hand. We take a piece of external 'evidence' about ourselves, and we run with it:

> ❝I have put on a lot of weight since the accident and I'm so immobile now that I can hardly get round the block let

alone to the gym four times a week like I used to. It gets me down. I feel less attractive, I can't fit into anything and I feel like people are dismissing me now in a way they never did when I was slim. I feel less of a person. 9

Shazia, 46, was knocked over by a car

Your body might have changed because of your health problem – possibly radically. It doesn't matter whether the changes are visible or hidden, they will affect how you feel about yourself.

Here are some ways that body changes can affect your life:

- Your social life:

  6 I don't want to go to my sister's wedding because of my weight gain. 9

  Shazia

- Your work life:

  6 My speech is slurred. Since so much of my work involves speaking in meetings, giving presentations and talking on the phone, I don't think I can do it any more. I'm considering early retirement. 9

  Julia, 56, had a stroke

- Your family life:

  6 I used to take my kids swimming every Saturday, but I hate showing my scars. My daughter says no one is looking at me, but I feel visible and vulnerable and I hate it. 9

  Luke, 44, had heart valve surgery

- Your sex life:

> ❝Even though my consultant says it won't, I can't stop worrying that sex will bring on another heart attack, so I haven't had sex with my wife for a year. I'm not the strong, healthy man she married. I think she isn't attracted to me any more anyway.❞
>
> **Jamie, 52, had a heart attack**

Finding ways to cope with your changed body takes time. Some of this is a matter of riding it out – scars fade, hair grows back, the weight might come off, or go back on. But often the timescale is months (sometimes years) rather than weeks.

In the meantime, in order to feel a lot better, you could try these coping strategies:

1 Talk about it – to family, friends, support groups, or more-anonymous phone lines or online contacts. When you are unhappy with your body it is easy to feel isolated, but talking can really help. Maybe the changes are not as huge as they feel (you may not look as different as you think; your partner may well still find you attractive). It is also possible that the changes that seem huge to you are far less obvious to others. If you can talk to people who have been through similar experiences, the relief can be huge. Being understood can boost your confidence tenfold. You may even get practical tips to make life easier.

2 Let yourself care. You might be relieved to have survived, and grateful to the medical team, and thankful for everything you have, but at the same time it's still reasonable to care about your appearance and how your body functions. It isn't frivolous or vain. How you feel about your body affects how you feel about yourself. Body image is not skin-deep.

3 Tackle avoidance. Facing your changed body is hard. It can, for example, be frightening to look under the bandages for the first time, or face your changed body in the mirror. It is therefore easy to get into the habit of avoidance. But if you can make yourself face these visible changes (perhaps start with glimpses, and build up the time you spend looking at them) the fear or squeamishness, or upset, will gradually fade. Confidence is catching – if you are OK about your body, others will be too.

Body image and your social life

If your physical changes are obvious, and you are afraid of how others will react, it can help to think through, in advance, a few coping strategies.

Prepare answers If you are worried that you'll face awkward questions, you could prepare a list of answers (write them down if that helps) so that you are confident that you will be able to cope when people say things. You can also take it very slowly; for example, at first you could go out with a close friend for support, and start with a small group for a short time. Build up gradually. As your confidence grows, socialising will seem like far less of an ordeal.

> ❛Children ask direct questions – and it used to freak me out. I'd clam up, go red, stutter. Then I decided I had to face this, head on. I got myself a tartan leg. My favourite trick is to take it off and hand it to kids. They love it, and laughter is a great ice-breaker.❜
>
> **Fergus, 45, amputee**

Use relaxation techniques One of the simplest and least obtrusive techniques for releasing tension is slowed breathing. After you breathe in, hold your breath for a moment, then breathe out slowly. Make sure that your out-breath is longer than your in-breath. It can help to purse your lips as if you're breathing out down a straw, and to notice your shoulders dropping and your muscles relaxing.

Think about how it went Try to be as balanced as you can, because there will be Thought Traps ready to jump up and tell you 'it was a bloody disaster'. Was it really? You may have felt hideously self-conscious, but did anyone say anything you couldn't handle? If it really was tough, it was a hurdle – and you got through it. Ask yourself what you've learned from this outing – see if you can think of things that might make it easier next time.

Accepting the new you

In a 1920 review of convalescence services for American soldiers injured in the First World War, a US doctor described the impact of serious injury on the soldiers' lives. 'The labourer enters the army, loses a leg or two, and by and by returns to his home not as a crippled labourer but as a skilled artisan, who now may with his head in a day earn more than with his legs in a week.' These words are quite shocking. But there is a message of hope here. What has happened to you might feel brutal. You may not want this 'new you' at all. But a huge part of regaining confidence is simply to accept that this has happened. You are where you are.

Colin, who lost his driving licence after his stroke, was at an all-time low, but he has managed to rebuild his confidence, independence and self-esteem.

⁶It took a while, but I gradually dropped the idea that I had to be driving to be living. Eventually I found out about a mobility scooter, and got one – from Denmark – 18 months after my stroke. It's been fantastic. I love having a vehicle again. It's given me the freedom to get out. Nowadays, I can

go with my wife to the supermarket, load up the heavy bags onto the scooter and take them home for her. I feel useful again. I'm not the same, but I am still me. ❜

* * * * *

No one is expecting you to forget about who you were before this happened to you. Sometimes you will feel sad, or angry or upset. But you can get yourself to the stage where you accept this new you – and enjoy it. This might be hard to believe right now, but it can – and will – happen if you take this chapter seriously.

In 1802 a French doctor, J.A.B. Fourcade, writing about convalescence, placed an emphasis upon 'light and air as aids to returning health'. Games and 'amusements' were recommended as promoting 'the tranquil spirit necessary for recovery'.

Colin was lost and angry for a long time. He was devastated, but eventually he found that tranquil spirit: he went outside, he made the most of 'light and air', he found his own 'amusements' – a puppy and a local bowls club. Above all, he recognised his own achievements. He worked out a new way to live, feel confident and be happy. So can you.

NOTES FOR CARERS

'We are not all made alike, we cannot be all giants in strength, and perhaps if you are weak in body you may have a more finely formed mind, a soul that though easily cast down can enjoy more in one hour than others more vigorously formed can in a week.'

Medicus, *Girls Own Paper***, 1880/1**

If someone you love loses their confidence, it can be very unsettling. It can change how you behave with each other – and it may catapult you into unexpected and unfamiliar roles. Again, the key for you, as the carer, is to stay calm and solid yourself. Here's how:

1 **Give it time** It can take a long time to adapt to change. Everyone is different, but in general, think in terms of months, or even years, rather than days or weeks.

2 **Let them talk about the loss and changes** It's tempting to challenge or 'reason' with people when they say unconfident things. When you care about someone, you want to 'solve' it for them. You want to *make* them feel better. You are not going to be able to do this for your loved one, but you can help them do it for themselves by listening to their sadness and loss and then (clearly but briefly) putting your point of view across. Don't expect them to believe or accept your perspective right away – they have to learn to believe this themselves.

3 **Show them how you feel about them** Don't just tell them in words that you think they're still valuable. Find ways to show them. Seek out their company/advice/talents/skills. Have a conversation and a laugh with them. Thank them for this. You could even put it in writing with a thank-you letter, email, text or note.

4 **Be honest about how you feel** It is OK to admit when it's difficult for you. But, equally, try to acknowledge any pleasure or advantage (however small!) that you discover in your new roles.

5 **Let them achieve things** Confidence comes from setting goals, achieving them, and recognising the achievement. You can really help by encouraging them to do this – reminding them of their achievements, demonstrating how far they've come, helping them to set further goals.

❝ Sally was still somewhat disabled when she got home after her stroke rehabilitation. But it was only at her follow-up a year later that her consultant measured her progress and pointed out to me that Sal was 62, not 92, and could do more than I thought. Since then, whenever I get "over considerate" she reminds me of this and I take a step back. It is lovely, she's nearly back to her old self. 〞

Alan, 68, husband of Sally

SIX

THE REST CURE

FATIGUE AND WHAT TO DO ABOUT IT

'After serious illness, medical or surgical, the patient,
before a completed convalescence is possible, must have
recovered from a condition of relative disorganisation of
the nervous system, both mental and motor.'

Dr John Bryant, *Convalescence*, 1927

In the late 1800s an American neurologist called Silas Weir
Mitchel (popularly known as 'Dr Diet and Dr Quiet'), devised
a 'rest cure' for Victorian 'hysterics' including the novelists
Virginia Woolf and Charlotte Perkins Gilman. These poor
women were subjected to six to eight weeks of total bed-rest,
constant force-feeding with fatty, milk-based foods, a ban on
reading, writing or speaking, and absolute isolation from
friends and family.

Clearly, this sort of thing is not going to work today. But it
is worth taking fatigue seriously. Think, for a moment, about
mild illnesses that you've had – throat infections, food poison-
ing, a bad cold. The chances are you felt listless for quite a while
afterwards. Even being mildly ill can bring on fatigue. It is
hardly surprising, then, that after a major health crisis fatigue
can be a serious issue – lasting weeks, months or even longer.

Fatigue is the burglar in your house: it is sneaky and very
hard to catch and tackle. But all the time it is stealing from
you – your *joie de vivre*, your get up and go, your capacity to
act and make decisions. Fatigue may not be life threatening,
but it is a huge barrier to feeling better, both emotionally and

physically. The good news is that you can do a lot to manage and relieve fatigue. But if you want to catch that burglar, you do have to take it seriously.

What is fatigue?

It might be best to start with what it's not. Fatigue is not a sign of weakness or inadequacy. It is nothing to do with getting older. And it may not be anything to do with sleep.

> Fatigue is a deep, pervasive and profound tiredness that impacts on many basic daily tasks and is not always relieved by sleep. It is a medically recognised after-effect of health problems.

Fatigue is more common, and lasts longer than any other post-surgical symptom. Up to 90 per cent of women experience fatigue after a hysterectomy. Over half of those who have a heart attack or heart surgery are fatigued several months later. And between 30 and 80 per cent of stroke patients are still feeling fatigue a year after their stroke. Fatigue is also the most common side effect of cancer treatment. In other words, if you are feeling fatigued after a health crisis, you are pretty normal.

❝I recovered quickly from my heart surgery. I was out of hospital within a week and back in the office three days later, but then this wall of exhaustion hit me. It was like nothing I'd ever experienced before. My mind just seized up and my body gave in. I felt like I couldn't move or think. I called my wife to collect me, went home, and eventually realised that I had a long road ahead.❞

Euan, 59, had a heart attack

Why does fatigue happen?

The rather poetic idea of fatigue as a 'disorganisation' of mind and body – outlined in the quote at the beginning of the chapter – really isn't as outdated as it sounds. When something serious happens to our bodies there are after-effects such as:

- Shock
- Ongoing pain/discomfort
- Medication side effects
- Lack of exercise/muscle loss
- Dietary or appetite changes
- Low mood
- Worries
- Disturbed sleep

All of these can lead to fatigue. Fatigue springs from a complex web of interacting factors:

The body's healing response When something happens to it, your body's healing response kicks in automatically. This brings a strong biological need to retreat and 'lick your wounds' – you're meant to crawl into your cave, pull a boulder across the entrance and stay there until you are strong enough to face the sabre-toothed tigers again.

Medical after-effects Many medications have side effects that include fatigue. The after-effects of anaesthesia can also last a surprisingly long time.

Immobility After a period of lying in bed you lose muscle strength. You might find it hard to sleep, or feel more breathless when you move, or have less appetite or be coping with ongoing pain. All of these things directly impact on your energy levels.

Emotional factors It is very common to feel down after a serious health problem. Low mood goes hand in hand with low energy. You may also feel more anxious than usual – anxiety can drain your energy, sometimes profoundly.

The fatigue rollercoaster

Fatigue rarely feels the same day in day out. A healthy person's energy levels fluctuate during the average day or week and it works the same way when you've had a health problem. The difference is that the energy swings may feel more extreme now.

You probably have a very sensitive energy 'radar' at the moment. You're more aware of your energy levels, and the peaks and troughs seem much bigger and less controllable than they did before your health problem.

When you do have some energy, the temptation is to try to get everything done – you get up, fire off emails, walk the dog, go to the supermarket, unload the shopping into a cupboard that you realise needs cleaning, clean the cupboard, sort out the messy shelves, fill in a form that you have been meaning to fill in for ages, take it to the Post Office, come home, cook – and collapse. For the next two days – more maybe – you are unable to do a thing. This is the fatigue rollercoaster.

When you go through this it is easy to think that your life is going to be ruled, from now on, by your unpredictable energy levels. You start to feel out of control. You can't plan; you can't get things done. This is distressing and frustrating.

⸾I had my stroke 13 months ago and I have made a pretty good recovery though I still have some left-sided weakness. But what I can't abide is the way in which I never know how much energy I am going to have from one day to the next. One day I find simple daily tasks like getting dressed, doing the ironing, deciding what to cook completely fine, whereas another day they can wipe me out. This not knowing how I will feel is holding me back. I am no longer a reliable person, I can no longer guarantee to be able to do things. ❯

Kavita, 42, had a stroke

The silence around fatigue

Although fatigue is one of the most common side effects of ill health, it gets very little attention at follow-up appointments – either from health professionals or their patients.

There are many reasons for this:

1 It's not easy to talk about it

Fatigue can be very difficult to describe. Many people don't feel able to 'bother' the doctor with vague complaints about tiredness. It is very common to (wrongly) assume that nothing can be done, so there's no point mentioning it. There might also be a sense of shame or inadequacy. 'What is wrong with me?' is a common thought. 'Other people bounce back, why can't I?'

❮ I should be full of energy, but I feel like an old man much of the time. I don't talk about it much because I don't want to sound like I'm whingeing or pathetic, but then I end up making excuses not to do things. I feel very alone. ❯

Tomasz, 32, had meningitis

2 Loved ones just don't get it

'I'm tired' doesn't really do it justice. Friends and family can therefore struggle to make sense of your fatigue. They may avoid mentioning how tired you seem because they don't want to make you feel worse. Or they may brush it off ('Oh, you'll soon bounce back'). They may try to explain it away ('You're not a spring chicken any more, you know'). They may even get irritated ('Oh, come on, you can do this!'). The general sense is bafflement. You're supposed to be getting better – why aren't you your old self?

> ❝I don't understand why it is so difficult for Judy to get up and going again – it is months since the operation. I feel like she's just given up.❞
> **Rob, husband of Judy, 61 who had a knee replacement**

3 Doctors seem too busy

Using your short appointment with the doctor to discuss fatigue may not feel like a good use of their limited time. Fatigue gets very little airtime in the information leaflets handed to patients as they leave hospital. It may only appear briefly as a topic in rehabilitation programmes. Indeed, research shows that many follow-up consultations simply don't address fatigue at all. Doctors may assume you're going to bring it up if it's a problem, and that the 'How have things been?' is enough of a prompt if you want to talk. Other members of a multi-disciplinary medical team – nurses, physiotherapists, occupational therapists, speech therapists, psychologists – can do this too. Sometimes medical professionals assume that someone else has asked you about fatigue, or that you'd raise it (assertively) if it were a problem. The consultation can therefore pass by without addressing the issue that's really holding you back.

> ❝I thought it was something to do with me, personally, not coping. I didn't feel able to really talk about it, even though it was a huge issue for me. I had so many other, seemingly more pressing issues and fatigue wasn't going

to kill me. If I ever said I felt tired, people would just look at me blankly, as if to say 'that's the least of your worries', so pretty early on I stopped saying it.

Chris, 52, who spent a month in intensive care after a car accident

Fatigue management

The great news is that fatigue can be tackled really effectively. There are three basic steps to managing your fatigue:

1 Talk (assertively) to your medical team: be honest, tell them how the fatigue is affecting your life and emotions, get their advice on strategies, ask about possible medication tweaks.

2 Make resting a habit.

3 Adopt the three Ps: Prioritise, Plan and Pace yourself.

Step 1: talk to your team

Before you make the appointment, put aside fears of 'whingeing'. Everyone wants you to recover. Fatigue interferes with recovery – no matter what it is you are recovering from. Therefore, if fatigue is a problem, your medical team will want to know. Here are some things to investigate with your team.

Is there a medical cause?

A medical consultation on fatigue is really a process of doctor detective work. The following factors could contribute to fatigue:

Anaemia If your red blood cells are not transporting oxygen around your body efficiently, physical actions involve more effort – and fatigue sets in.

Medications Fatigue is a major side effect of many drugs. Sometimes the interaction between medications is to blame. Your doctor may be able to tweak your medication in order to improve your energy levels.

Diet Yours may be missing some essential energy-boosting nutrients. Some people find that dietary advice from a registered dietician makes a huge difference to fatigue management. Your doctor may be able to refer you to someone reliable.

Depression Fatigue is a common feature of depression (most people with depression feel fatigued, although not all people with fatigue are depressed). If you feel low, fatigue can be a huge issue. One of the best ways of tackling low mood or depression is to get fatigue under control. Sometimes, a doctor may decide that a short course of antidepressants will lift your mood enough so that you can put fatigue (and depression) management strategies into practice.

Your body's limitations You will have lost muscle bulk if you spent any more than a couple of days in bed, and to get your energy back you'll need to build your muscle bulk back up. (See Chapter 10.)

Even if, in the end, there isn't an appropriate medical treatment for your fatigue, your medical team will be able to reassure you that it is OK for you to follow the suggestions in this book, so do talk to them about fatigue.

Step 2: make resting a habit

⟨It becomes excessively important to avoid the occurrence of fatigue. This may be most easily and perhaps best accomplished by a system of five minutes rests (in the reclining position) for each thirty minutes of effort. It should be noted that if the patient eats sitting up during the first few days the fatigue factors are doubled. To a certain extent this special factor may be overcome by insistence upon a glass of water and twenty minutes of flat rest before the meals are served. ⁹

Dr John Bryant, *Convalescence*, 1927

Nobody is going to insist that you lie down at dinnertime, but the idea of getting a balance between activity and rest worked in the 1920s and works today. In fact, there is now a body of modern scientific studies showing that this is a highly effective way to tackle fatigue.

Most of us rest when we feel worn out. But, with fatigue, you have to learn to rest before you're pooped.

How to rest

It's tempting to skip the rest bit, even when you're deliberately trying to pace yourself. Rest can be surprisingly hard to do, unless you're exhausted and have no choice but to collapse. The very idea of rest can actually be a bit scary for some people. It can feel like a reminder of being bedbound. Or it might seem like a sign of weakness or failure to recover. You might worry that resting is somehow wimpy, lazy or self-indulgent – or, at the very least, boring. It might feel like a sign of ageing, of reduced abilities, or of all you've lost. If you find yourself resisting the idea of rest, it might be worth asking yourself why – what is it about rest that you don't like?

❛Rest feels like wasted time, time when I could be out doing things, looking after my animals. My wife has to hide my boots to stop me going out again at night. This bloody accident has forced me to stop in at home and I hate it, it makes me feel useless. But I now try to use this damned resting to build up my determination to get back to where I was before. 9

Adrian, 58, had abdominal surgery after a farming accident

Other people can be unhelpful. Throwaway comments such as 'Oh, what I wouldn't give for a chance to put my feet up like you', 'You're living a life of luxury', 'Am I your slave now?' can be hard to handle, particularly if, like Adrian, you are already feeling frustrated and vulnerable.

This has long been the case. In fact, Sheila Pim wrote in her *Convalescents' Handbook* in 1943 that, 'Convalescence looks good enough to the outsider. A lazy life with people waiting on you hand and foot, and nothing to do but eat and sleep. In spite of this convalescents are known to bite the hands that feed them ... it is not really their fault, for they are going through an awkward transition period.'

If you don't rest, your transition period will stay awkward. You will remain strapped in the fatigue rollercoaster. It therefore seems more sensible to accept the scientifically tested idea of rest – and feel better.

TIP

Time-limit your rest

Endless rest is just inactivity. You are trying to become more active, not less. So, you have to be as strict about rest times as you are about getting up and moving around. Set a timer for 15 or 30 minutes (or whatever time period you are using) when you sit down to rest. Get up and do things again as soon as rest time is over.

To nap or not to nap

Rest time doesn't actually mean taking a nap, although it's easy to confuse the two. In fact, naps might be best avoided, as they can interrupt night-time sleep (see Chapter 7, page 195). If you do nap, make it planned and brief – not longer than 15 minutes (especially if you struggle with sleep at night). To avoid napping at rest times it helps not to be in bed. In fact, during a rest you don't have to be totally immobile. You can read, stretch, have a cup of tea, do a crossword or chat on the phone (to an undemanding friend) – these are all 'restful' things to do. The key to rest is purely to do less physically strenuous things, so as to balance out your activity.

TIP

Call it something else

If the word 'rest' makes you edgy, try renaming it: 'muscle recovery time', 'taking a break', 'catch-up time', 'quiet time', 'wind-down time'. Remember that athletes build rest into their schedules and know that it is as valuable as their exercise time.

Get moving!

Exercise is a vital part of fatigue management. But wait – you've just been told for pages and pages to rest. Now you're being told to move more! How could this be?

Your body has been through the mill – your muscles are likely to be weaker, you may be physically damaged, and you are almost certainly less fit than you were before this health problem. Exercise will give you more, not less, energy, whatever age or stage you are at. The trick is to do the right amount for you, at the right times, building up what you do slowly, and balancing it with rest. (See Chapter 10 for tips on how to do this.)

You probably already know you should exercise daily, but maybe you've told yourself that, because of what's happened to you, this advice doesn't really apply to you right now because you're so tired. Well, it does. Activity, however much you can manage, will rebuild your lost muscle mass, release endorphins ('feel-good' hormones), increase your fitness and – yes – reduce fatigue.

Step 3: adopt the three Ps

There are three key strategies for managing all this resting and activity. They are to:

1 Prioritise: what you need or want to get done (you can't do it all).

2 Plan: how you'll achieve this.

3 Pace yourself: be realistic about how much you can do, and when.

Strategy one: prioritise

The idea of having to make decisions about what you can and can't do may be very hard, almost painful. But it is vital. Try to 'weed' your life:

1 Write a list of all the tasks that you have been trying to juggle; for example, 'looking after myself – looking after others – managing the home – doing my job – hobbies – seeing friends'.

2 Work out which ones you can (temporarily) drop – or at least delegate. Think about the tasks that are troublesome or too difficult for the time being. Write them down. These questions will help you to establish which tasks are most meaningful to you, and what you can change:

- What tasks make me feel good about myself and/or feel particularly personal? (For example, seeing family, doing charity work, going to an art class.)

❛I used to work for a theatre design company, hand-sewing all their props and costumes. But after my first episode of surgery I realised I couldn't cope with the pressure of deadlines and such exacting requirements. I was medically retired from work but set up a little business from home teaching people how to sew. I love it, I meet people, I feel useful, but I can control how much I do. As a teacher I don't have to do so much of the sewing, so my joints don't suffer as much.❜

Geethi, 50, has rheumatold arthritis

- What tasks absolutely have to be done by me? (For example, the school run, the accounts, a hospital follow-up.) Think carefully about this – does it really have to be you or is there someone else who could do it? (And might they even enjoy doing it?)

❛I used to do all the cooking but when I first got home from hospital my partner set up a family "Come Dine With Me" so each person was responsible for cooking supper one night a week. It took the pressure off me and was fun for the whole family. We still do it about one week a month. We also order in pizza more often than before my injury.❜

Lauren, 48, had burns treatment on her leg

- What tasks are less important or meaningful to you? Are there chores that could be ditched or at least reduced? (For example, ironing all the sheets, vacuuming every day, cooking all your meals from scratch.) If you can't ditch them, can you reduce or alter them, or get someone else to do them for you? (If so, who?) This might involve lowering your standards, but it can be a huge relief.

❝I love gardening but have always hated mowing the lawn, so now I forget perfection – I leave the lawn for as long as I can and then pay the lad from next door to come and do it for me.❞

Graham, 60, had coronary bypass surgery

- What tasks use up a lot of physical or mental energy? Do you really need to do these things now? If you have to do them – is there a way to make them easier?

❝I went back to work before I could type again so I used voice recognition software for a bit. There were some ludicrous mistakes, but I got my work done.❞

Sylvia, 39, had hand surgery

The point here is that you can't just pick everything back up and carry on where you left off. That will lead you right back onto the rollercoaster. You have to let some things go, even if it hurts. You can then focus on those that are most important to you.

Strategy two: plan

'Weighing up the number of things one wants in the course of an afternoon against the nuisance of carrying too much luggage about the garden, it often seems too much trouble to go out after all. If you have no summerhouse ... you might perhaps consecrate a suitcase to garden occupations, or better still a tea

trolley. The fit up could include: a small cushion, a light rug that folds up small, a sunshade, a fan, cigarettes and matches. If you are a non-smoker you will sometimes need to make a smoke to keep off midges. A writing pad and pencil, books – small handbooks to help you identify birds or butterflies. A magnifying glass for looking at beetles. A tin of biscuits. These are for the birds as well as you.'

Sheila Pim, *Handbook for Convalescents*, 1943

Pim is right: without planning, an activity – even just going into the garden – can quickly become overwhelming when you are battling fatigue. Planning your life may sound fussy and – yes – frankly exhausting. But you'd be surprised how much you plan already without knowing it – anything from setting your morning alarm, to making a coffee date with a friend. Planning is not a ridiculous idea, you just have to up the ante a bit when you are fatigued. Try to make a weekly plan:

Geeky types can use clever electronic devices or spreadsheets for planning, but even the back of an envelope will do. The main thing is to see your week planned out in front of you. You are aiming to create a balanced week, where bouts of activity are interspersed with episodes of rest. Try to make sure that you don't schedule too many activities in one day – juggle and cancel things, if necessary or possible, so that you can spread out your activity.

1 Sit down on a Sunday night for half an hour and look at the week ahead. List everything you have to do – include both big and small tasks (load the washing machine/book the bar mitzvah/see the doctor).

2 Note down which are routine tasks (weekly supermarket shop/drive kids to school/walk the dog) and which are unusual (dinner with friends/hospital appointment/major work presentation).

3 Juggle and tweak to find a balance. If Monday is packed, can you move a meeting to Tuesday? Can you ask a friend to give you a lift to the swimming pool rather than the tiring bus ride on Friday? Can you do the shopping on Thursday not Wednesday, as you have six other things already on Wednesday? Can you break any tasks down? Do they all need to be done in one go? Can you do your tax return over a couple of weeks rather than all in one weekend? Does the car journey to visit friends have to be done in rush hour without a break? Think about anything that can help you (a wheeled shopping bag, a relaxation app on your smart phone?)

4 Plan when and how you will integrate rests into your day – at home on the sofa? In the supermarket café? In the first-aid room for 15 minutes twice a day at work? Schedule them, and plan how long you'll rest for. If you don't timetable rests into each day, the rollercoaster can speed up and make it very hard for you to stop for a break.

TIP

Longer-term plans – how to avoid unwanted pressure

Making longer-term plans might feel hard right now, and that's OK. The trouble is that people close to you may not get this. They may become a bit over-excited when you start feeling better and plan all sorts of treats and surprises for you. If this sounds great then that's wonderful, but for many people this can feel like a pressure. 'I have to be better by January to fly to India!' may not be a relaxing thought. You may therefore have to explain to loved ones that you just aren't ready to make long-term plans yet. Explain that you are trying to focus on medium- and short-term plans for now – week by week. This will let them down gently but also show them that it's not that you're just doing 'nothing'.

HOW TO REST AT WORK

Resting at work may seem like a preposterous idea. But it might be essential for you right now. Obviously, it can be incredibly hard to achieve. This is why you should start by talking to your human resources department and/or your boss about your fatigue. Explain that fatigue is a response to what you've been through – a medical issue. Explain that you are implementing strategies to tackle it. Try to explore ways you can make your working day less tiring – for example could you time your working day to avoid the rush hour? Is working from home one day a week feasible? Could you work flexi hours, teleconference, or actually take your lunch break? Could you split your lunch break into a short break in the morning, midday and afternoon? Is there a first-aid room where you could lie down for 15 minutes twice a day? Only you can know what is feasible for you and your workplace, but rest at work is only likely to happen if you make it official. Making it official will stop you feeling 'guilty', and will tackle the fear that people will think you are 'shirking'. Fatigue management at work will allow you to be far more productive. You will have fewer sick days. You will be a better team member. This is not a luxury!

❝It was a really difficult decision for me, but a couple of months after my cancer treatment I was so tired I realised I could not go back to work full time or do the same things. I'm a vet and I'd been working out on farms with large animals, but I just didn't have the energy to manage that. I sat down with the partners in the practice and we agreed that I'd go back five mornings a week but would stay in the practice seeing small animals for the first six months and then we'd review. I'm coming up to the review and I'm pretty confident that I can build up my hours closer to full time, as I now know how to prioritise and plan, and I can see that rest periods really work. ❞

Billy, 32, had testicular cancer

Plan for overload

You may look at your week and see a day that's just going to be a nightmare of over-activity and there's nothing you can do about it. The temptation at this point is to think, 'This planning business just isn't working – my life isn't like that!' But even the busiest people can plan. The trick is to plan ways to cope with setbacks or overloads.

Here's how:

1. Look at the rest of your day or week; see if you can find any opportunities – however small – for a break or rest. Can you change or drop anything at all?
2. Ask for help. This is easier said than done, but think about anyone who could help you get through this tricky period – you may find people more willing than you'd think.
3. Watch your Thought Traps – you may catastrophise ('This is never going to work!') or put on 'filter glasses' ('I haven't planned my week at all!') or label yourself ('I'm hopeless – I've totally failed in this planning thing, I knew I would'). (See page 174.)

Sometimes you simply have to get through the overload – recognise that it's not forever, then start planning sensibly again when you can.

Strategy three: pace yourself

With fatigue, your energy levels tend to fluctuate during the day – sometimes wildly. To tackle this, it helps to break up your activities and goals into manageable chunks and balance them with rests. The tricky thing is working out what is 'manageable' for you. As Sheila Pim told her 1940s' convalescents: 'To rest when you are tired brings you up to where you were before, but to rest when you are not particularly tired ... charges the battery.'

Try this: charge your battery

Try to identify the tasks that particularly tire you out. One simple example might be vacuum cleaning the house. On bad (fatigued) days you can only vacuum for 15 minutes before you're exhausted. Now, think about what would be easy for you even on one of these bad days – say, 5 minutes of vacuuming. To find a reasonable target for this activity you need to aim for somewhere between those two times. In this case, you'd set yourself 10 minutes of vacuuming time before it's time to rest. You can use this model for any task, big or small.

Limit yourself to your target time even when you're having a good day and feel you 'could' ('should'?) do more. Doing this stops you getting back on the rollercoaster – doing too much, then crashing.

❝I had my stroke while we were building a conservatory. I was left with a very weak right arm and hand. The building work was probably the best therapy there was, and the most frustrating. From the demolition I had over 2,000 Victorian bricks, all of which needed the mortar cleaning off. I started off left-handed, and managed about six an hour. Mental arithmetic meant the job at that rate would have taken many months even if I did it full time. I found eventually I could hold the trowel in my left hand and steady it with the right, then I progressed to the trowel in my right hand steadied with my left, and eventually in my right hand more or less unaided. The transformation took about two months.❞

Tim, 55, had a stroke

Tackling mental fatigue

Fatigue after illness or injury is not always just physical. The feelings of exhaustion can also affect your concentration, decision-making or memory. This might explain why Victorian and Edwardian convalescents so loved 'Coca Wine'. This feel-good tonic 'for fatigue of mind and body' contained both cocaine and alcohol. No wonder they felt temporarily uplifted. These days, mental fatigue is just as common after ill health – but people tend to suffer in silence. This can be really distressing.

> My memory changed after my hysterectomy. I am a counsellor and I used to be able to remember sessions verbatim, but after my surgery I couldn't do that any more. I had to learn a new way of remembering things. I had to take notes, I had to develop memory techniques, I had to maintain my confidence. Luckily, I had a very understanding supervisor. I was able to cut down to part time at work and my family were supportive. It was a difficult time, but actually I think I have become a better counsellor because of it. I think more carefully and make more connections.
>
> **Nicola, 54, had a hysterectomy**

Some research shows that cognitive ability (things like concentration, memory or attention) can decline after surgery – both major and more minor surgical procedures. This is usually temporary but this 'brain fog' can still last weeks, months, or even in a small number of people, up to one or two years.

How to tackle brain fog

- Anxiety definitely affects how sharp your mind feels. If you cannot find your car keys and you begin to panic and think that you really are losing your mind, try to calmly remind yourself that this is OK, it's not a sign of anything sinister – this is temporary.

- Write notes. Carry a notebook or smartphone with a notes section, in which you jot down thoughts and reminders to yourself as they occur to you – it's like carrying an ongoing to-do list with you.

- Create a structure. If it feels like you are always losing your keys or your phone or bag, set up a solution: get yourself a peg board where you keep keys, and make yourself hang them on it whenever you finish using them. Or put a chair by the front door and keep your bag on it. Pop an instruction list on the door of the fridge to remind yourself of the mundane tasks and appointments you can't forget (bins out Tuesday, unplug TV before bed, flu jab appointment Thursday).

- Have a mental workout – read books or newspapers. If your vision is restricted, listening to the radio news or audio books is just as good. You could join a book club, or talk to a bookish friend – talking about intellectual things helps too! Watch a TV quiz that interests you and test yourself against the contestants. Or, try puzzles – jigsaws, sudoku, code words or crosswords.

- Exercise your body. Research shows that physical exercise such as walking, yoga or sports can protect against the onset of memory difficulties in older adults and appears to slow the rate of disease progression in dementia-type illnesses. Exercise (planned and paced) certainly can't hurt if you're feeling 'foggy brained'.

Tackling fatigued thoughts

Our thoughts drive our behaviour – they are hunched there, like a madman gripping the steering wheel, making us turn this way or that. When you push yourself too far and too fast, there are thoughts lurking behind your actions, their foot pressed on the accelerator – or the brake pedal (stopping you from having a go, from trying something out). Part of tackling fatigue is to recognise the Thought Traps that go with it. Common fatigue Thought Traps include:

- Unrealistic/harsh expectations: 'I should be able to do this myself', 'I must not ask for help', 'Having a rest is just lazy', 'No one else can do the job as well as I can', 'My home should be spotless.'

- All-or-nothing thinking: 'If I can't finish the job today there is no point in starting it', 'If I ask for help, I'll be dependent forever.'

- Mind-reading: 'They think I'm sitting around doing nothing', 'I have bothered people enough; they won't want to come out for a walk with me', 'I can't ask for help, she's so busy it'd be such an imposition.'

- Fortune-telling: 'I am never going to feel like myself again', 'My life is going to be restricted by this bloody pacing forever.'

- Catastrophising: 'If I don't manage to get my energy back, my life is over', 'I feel worse today – this programme is just not working.'

If you catch yourself falling into Thought Traps such as 'If I can't finish the job today, there is no point in starting it', it is important to put your wig on and lay out your 'case for the defence'.

Build your 'case for the defence'

What's the evidence? Is it possible that if you take more time and thought over this job the result might actually be better than if you rush it? Is this job really urgent? Can you get some of it done today, and the rest later? Are you underestimating how much time you have? Even if you have to take breaks and stop for rests, can you still get this job done?

What are the 'mitigating circumstances'? You have been ill and you are fatigued, you will not be able to do as much as before. But if you can start this task you will have evidence that you are rebuilding your strength and abilities.

Is thinking like this fair or helpful? Who says the job has to be done today? Is there a genuine deadline, or are you pressurising yourself unfairly? Is thinking in all-or-nothing terms going to help you to implement fatigue management strategies or instead keep you strapped into the fatigue rollercoaster? If the pesky colleague who is after your job was to say to you, 'Don't bother to start that job, if you can't get it done today' wouldn't you defend yourself? If you can defend yourself to them you can also defend yourself from your own harsh thoughts.

In days gone by, people understood that fatigue was a normal consequence of ill health and that it took time to overcome. But nowadays we have this bonkers idea that we'll leap off the surgeon's table or out of the sick bed and magically be full of beans – right away. This just isn't realistic. Overcoming fatigue can be a slow and frustrating process. It can be disheartening at times. Tim, who was building his conservatory brick by brick after his stroke, realised that he could not do it alone. He ended up employing a couple of local lads to help with the heavy work. But after around 18 months, he says,

> ❛I managed to install the new kitchen more or less unaided. It was difficult, but very little was real detailed work and . . . I took my time. I would do a bit and then stop for a cuppa. ❜

Tim found his physical restrictions tough, but he kept going:

> ❝I religiously did the arm and hand exercises I had been given by my physiotherapist and little by little I got stronger. I did my first detailed job in May this year. I made a large wooden jigsaw puzzle for my two-year-old granddaughter's birthday. She loves it.❞

* * * * *

If you stick with the strategies in this chapter, you will cope with fatigue far better than if you just wait and hope it will go away. If you manage your fatigue, you will feel able to face the world again. You may not be your 'old self' but you'll realise this new one is pretty good too.

NOTES FOR CARERS

'Almost every effect of over-exertion appears after, not during, such an exertion. It is the highest folly to judge of the sick, as is so often done, when you see them merely during a period of excitement.'

Florence Nightingale, *Notes on Nursing,* **1859**

Fatigue can be very confusing and frustrating for everyone involved. At the height of a health crisis it usually seems understandable, but then it lingers – and that can be unnerving, and at times even baffling. Here are some ways to cope when you are caring for someone with fatigue:

1 **Remind yourself that it's a 'real' condition** Fatigue is one of the most common and long-lasting medical consequences of illness or injury. The person you are caring for is not being awkward/difficult/lazy/a moaner.

2 **Talk to their health-care team** A discussion about the difficulties of fatigue might seem less awkward coming from you (but agree on this together before the appointment).

3 **Use the three Ps for yourself too** Building both rest and exercise into your life is absolutely vital for carers. Doing this will help your energy levels (caring for someone can be deeply sapping). It will also show your fatigued loved one that these strategies are feasible – and work.

4 **Agree on how you can help with their fatigue management** It is easy to feel like a nag ('Sit down!', 'Isn't it time for your exercise?', 'No, we can't do that, you have to rest', 'Did you really do 10 minutes on the exercise bike?'). You may feel crushed by the responsibility of constantly having to monitor someone (who perhaps doesn't want monitoring). You can become exhausted too. So, agree what you're going to help with – and how – and stick to your side of the bargain.

⟨To push or not to push, that was the question. After Alex finished his treatment it was incredibly hard to know what or how much he should be doing. He was tired so much of the time. He would try things, push too hard and then flake out. It was difficult and we got quite cross with each other. But he learnt at a support group about gradually building up his energy through exercise and pacing. Now we go shopping together but stop for breaks. He pushes the trolley and I carry the bags home. It takes planning but he is no longer exhausted all the time, and he can see that he is progressing. ⟩
Jack, 37, partner of Alex, 48, who had leukaemia

SEVEN

COUNTING SHEEP

SLEEP, AND HOW TO GET SOME

'Sleep is to be sought for above all things, and when it comes and lasts, recovery is almost sure.'

Le Roi Goddard Crandon and Albert Ehrenfried
***Surgical After Treatment*, 1912**

In days gone by, attitudes to convalescence had one thing in common: an obsession with sleep. In the *Girls Own Paper* (1888/9) a doctor columnist, Medicus, advised those who were struggling with sleep to exercise well during the day, ventilate the bedroom, eat only a light supper, and sleep on a 'hardish' mattress. Above all, he said, girlish invalids should avoid stimulation: 'You must not read silly novels,' he instructed, 'especially these pretty little stories of love and murder which are all too fashionable.'

He was at least partially right: the keys to good sleep are, indeed, to release tension, avoid over-stimulation and create a healthy sleep environment. It is virtually impossible to feel better if you are not getting enough sleep. Apart from anything else, sleep helps the body to heal. While you are asleep your body releases restorative antibodies and hormones to help you fight off illnesses and recuperate. Without good sleep, your body cannot produce enough of these protective and infection-fighting cells.

Sleep is, in fact, an instinctive response to many common illnesses. When you catch the flu your instinct is usually to curl up and sleep. Your clever body is telling you, loud and clear, how to feel better.

Emotionally, sleep is important too. If your nights are filled with long hours counting sheep, tossing and turning, or falling asleep only to wake in the wee hours, then sleep – or lack of it – can quickly become a source of deep stress. Stress is not good if you want to feel better.

Sleep problems cause all sorts of daytime problems, too, including tiredness, memory loss, difficulty concentrating, irritability and depression. Poor sleep can affect your sense of self, your academic or work life, your relationships – and your recovery.

Pain, movement problems, sedentary days, certain medications, worries and stresses can all interrupt sleep.

> ❝I woke up every hour of every night for the first fortnight after surgery. It was horrendous. I dreaded the nights but I was also affected during the day. I couldn't concentrate or remember things; at times I couldn't even hold a pretty basic conversation. I felt like I was being tortured. It's not nearly as bad now four months on, but even so, my sleep is not what it once was.❞
>
> **Vijay, 67, had a hip replacement**

What is surprising is how little we talk about sleep problems. This may be because they do not seem actively life-threatening. Indeed, if you have had complex medical problems involving hi-tech interventions, sleep issues can seem a bit basic. There is also a feeling that sleep will somehow sort itself out. It may, but it may also take a very long time to do so.

There is, in fact, a growing recognition in the medical world that sleep is vital for recovery. Recent studies, for example, have looked at patients in intensive care units (ICU), where sleep can be badly disrupted. Researchers have found that making simple changes to the ICU environment (such as reducing noise and light, and shortening the length of investigations at night) does not just improve the patients' sleep patterns, it also increases the speed and quality of the patients' recovery.

In short, if you want to feel better, sleep is not a luxury – it's an essential.

Do you have a sleep problem?

Sleep problems include:

- Difficulty getting off to sleep
- Waking in the night
- Struggling to get back to sleep during the night
- Early morning waking
- Waking up each day feeling unrested

If you are dissatisfied by the quantity and/or quality of your sleep on at least three nights a week for at least three months, you may have a sleep problem.

> ❝ For the first few weeks at home I was terrified about going to sleep – I think I was scared that if I closed my eyes I might never wake up. I stayed up late, I got my wife to stay up with me, I tried to tire myself out, I even tried sleeping in a chair instead of going to bed. My sleep became totally disrupted and so did my days. I was a mess. ❞
>
> **Gareth, 57, had a pulmonary embolism**

Many people think that beyond popping pills there isn't much you can do about sleep problems. Fortunately, that isn't true. Although it isn't easy to change sleep habits, it is possible. But before you try to solve your sleep problems, it is important to understand the basics about sleep.

Sleep disruption: the prime suspects

After a health problem, sleep can be disrupted for all sorts of reasons:

1 Body response to 'crisis': illness or injury can trigger changes to your hormones, metabolic rate, blood composition or the activity of the nervous system. These changes are all known to disrupt sleep.

2 Body's response to surgery: after surgery, the disruptions described above actually have a medical name, 'surgical stress response'. Doctors believe that the 'surgical stress response' disrupts sleep even more than anaesthesia (see box below).

3 Ongoing health issues: pain, fever, nausea, bladder weakness or other ongoing issues can all disrupt your sleep, as can a lack of physical activity.

4 Medications: these can affect your sleep patterns and quality.

5 Emotions: shock, fear, worry, confusion and uncertainty can create huge physical and mental tension, racing, intrusive thoughts and agitated behaviour – not the recipe for a good night's sleep.

SURGICAL STRESS RESPONSE

In one rather bizarre experiment, researchers put people under general anaesthetic for several hours without doing any surgery. They compared these patients' sleep patterns to the sleep patterns of patients who were put under anaesthetic but also had surgery. Those who had an anaesthetic without surgery had disrupted sleep for a night or two. But those who had surgery experienced sleep disruptions for one or two weeks afterwards. Studies also show that longer, more invasive surgery tends to disrupt a patient's sleep patterns more than minor surgery.

Your body clock

Your sleep patterns are strongly influenced by your 24-hour 'body clock' (also known as your 'circadian rhythms'). Your body clock encourages you to sleep when it is dark and wake up at sunrise. But when you have a health problem it is easy to develop unhelpful habits such as sleeping during the day and waking up during the night. These habits can disrupt your body clock, and stop you sleeping 'normally' when you want to.

What is 'normal' sleep?

Most of us think normal sleep is just a constant period of flat-out snoring. But there is actually a lot going on, physically and mentally, during sleep.

Falling asleep is a bit like turning a computer off. The computer doesn't instantly shut down like a light bulb. First, it has to log off, then it must close down all its systems one by one (and – yes – the older the computer, the longer it takes to close down). Your body does this too: you don't just 'shut down', you make a gradual transition from wakefulness to sleeping.

During sleep, you go through cycles of deep and light sleep. The periods of lightest sleep are called rapid eye movement (REM) sleep: these occur several times a night, including when you first fall asleep, and just before you wake up. REM sleep is when you dream.

A typical adult sleep pattern goes like this:

1 Feeling drowsy, nodding off, entering the sleep cycle (REM sleep)

2 Transition towards deeper sleep

3 Deep sleep

4 Deepest sleep

5 REM sleep (possibly waking up slightly)

6 Transition back to deeper sleep again

7 This REM/deep-sleep cycle continues throughout the night until you have your final REM cycle and wake up

The sleep cycle is like a staircase. The stages of light REM sleep are at the top, the deepest sleep is at the bottom and you go up and down this staircase several times a night. On average we all actually wake up during REM sleep at least twice a night. Most of us don't notice these wake ups; however, when your health is causing you problems – if you're conscious of pain, or stress, or discomfort – then you are more likely to notice these REM wake ups. It can also be harder to get back 'downstairs' to deep sleep afterwards.

AGE AND SLEEP

As we age, we naturally spend more time at the top of the staircase and less time in the deep and deepest stages of sleep (older people tend to have lighter and more broken sleep). On average, a person over 70 spends only 10 per cent of their sleep cycle in deepest sleep, compared to 30 per cent of the sleep cycle for a young adult.

How much sleep is enough?

How long is a piece of string? Our sleep requirements change with age: babies sleep for up to 18 hours a day, toddlers need long daytime naps and around 12 hours at night. Teenagers can shift towards 8 or 9 hours of sleep, but may start falling asleep later and waking later in the morning (or possibly afternoon). Adults get by on an average of 7–8 hours of sleep a night, but older adults may need only 5 or 6 hours (possibly with the odd daytime nap).

Sleep needs are not just about life stages, though. Margaret Thatcher famously ran Britain on four hours a night; Bill Clinton claimed to get by on five; Abraham Lincoln was known for his midnight insomniac strolls. One adult may feel rested and alert after just a few hours' sleep, whereas another may not be able to function without nine. But sleep is not a competitive sport. The only thing that matters is the outcome: whether or not you feel rested and able to function well. There is no law that says you have to get seven hours a night, or be sleeping like a baby at 4.30 am.

SLEEP MYTHS

It is easy to beat yourself up if you are sleeping badly and assume that your poor sleep is bound to (further) damage your health; however, your sleep may be better than you fear. The science is often very reassuring:

MYTH 'I had a bad night last night, so tonight I have to catch up on all that lost sleep.'

FACT Just getting a period of good-quality deep sleep – at some point in the night – is enough to restore your body and mind if you slept badly the night before.

MYTH 'I have to get eight hours a night or I won't function properly the next day.'

FACT The average adult needs 7–8 hours a night, but that's just an *average*. Individual needs vary widely (see above). Five or six hours could, in fact, be perfectly fine for you.

MYTH 'Sleep is only "good" if it is uninterrupted.'

FACT You do not have to sleep for one consistent block of time at night. Being awake for a bit in the middle of the night does not mean the rest of your sleep will not be restorative.

MYTH 'If I'm exhausted all day, it means I'm not getting enough sleep.'

FACT Feeling tired during the day may be nothing to do with night-time sleep – it may be fatigue, which sleep does not necessarily help (see Chapter 6).

Ways to sleep better

People who sleep well rarely give sleep a second thought, but those who don't can obsess on it endlessly. And the more you worry about not sleeping, the harder it is to sleep. You may also be worrying about other things too, or reliving bad memories.

> ❝The minute I lie down, everything that has happened comes flooding back and I know that I will be awake for hours. ❞
>
> **Maria, 36, had an ectopic pregnancy**

What you need is a way to stop worries and thoughts from sabotaging your sleep. Here are two ways to defuse thoughts and worries:

1 *Keep a notebook and pen by the bed*

Sometimes your thoughts get stuck on a loop. If you write them down, you no longer have to hold them in your head – your brain can let go. We all get light-bulb moments but when we wake up the next day it's gone. Your brain is cunning. It knows this can happen. So, it tries to outwit you. It keeps replaying the thought so that it won't get lost. This is why, when you toss and turn, you can't get certain thoughts out of your mind. Writing the thoughts in a notebook signals to your brain that it's OK – the thought is captured. Now you can sleep.

2 *Bomb disposal before (not in) bed*

Although some disrupted nights come out of the blue, many come after a difficult day or before a worrying appointment. Sometimes you can predict some of the worrying thoughts that are like little ticking bombs that will explode the moment you get into bed. The trick is to defuse and dispose of those bombs in advance. Try this bomb-disposal technique towards the end of the evening but before you start to wind down:

1 Write down the problem that is bothering you the most (or that you think is going to kick in when you go to bed).

2 Consider how you would solve that problem. Brainstorm a range of possible solutions, from the very sensible to the frankly bizarre.

3 When you can think of nothing else at all, look at what you've written and choose the most helpful solution.

4 Think about what you'd need to do in order to put this solution into practice – write that down too.

5 Once you have done this, stop writing. You have disposed of your bomb. You can put your notebook/computer/scrap of paper away and start to wind down (see 'Wind-down time', page 188).

6 When you get into bed, if the bomb starts ticking again, you can tell it to stop. It has been defused already, so it can't explode.

Bomb disposal may sound simplistic, but it works.

TIP

Tell yourself you don't need to sleep

This little trick can work miracles. First, remind yourself of the sleep facts (page 184). Tell yourself it's completely fine to be awake. You can be awake all night if you want. You can even instruct yourself categorically *not* to go to sleep – you're going to stay awake. This takes the pressure off. It's definitely worth a try on one of those nights when nothing else seems to be working (think about wise old Mary Poppins singing to the overexcited children 'stay awake, don't rest your head').

Relax your body

Victorian doctors mostly believed that insomnia was a physical problem, caused by things like blood flow problems or 'brain congestion'. Consequently, the Victorians generally advocated physical treatments for sleep problems. It is certainly true that sleep problems and physical tension are linked. Good sleep will only happen if your body is relaxed. The great news is that it is perfectly possible to relax the body. Here are three good ways to relax your body:

1 Slow breathing

This should almost always be your first port of call when tense. The basic idea is simply to breathe out for longer than you breathe in, thereby calming the body's stress response (see Chapter 2, page 48, for a full explanation)

Add-ons: add these three elements to your slow breathing to deepen the relaxation.

- Notice your shoulders: notice how your shoulders rise with your in-breath. Pay attention to your shoulders as they drop back down with the out-breath.

- Consciously relax: imagine the relaxed feeling from your out-breath spreading down your arms, down your body and out through your legs.

- Talk to yourself (in your mind): on the out-breath say a calming word: 'calm', 'relaxed', 'quiet', 'loose', 'warm', 'heavy', 'sleepy'. Try to imagine these feelings flowing through your body as you say the word. You can do a statement if that feels easier: 'I'm OK', 'I'm relaxed', 'I'm sleepy.'

2 Muscle squeeze–release

Tensing your muscles before you release them allows for a deeper physical release. Muscle squeeze–release is perfect when you are lying in bed feeling tense (or even before you get to this stage). (See Chapter 2, page 51, for how to do muscle squeeze–release.)

3 Visualisation

Try this after your slow breathing or muscle squeeze–release. Yes, you're right: visualisation is using your mind – but the mind can have a miraculously relaxing effect on the body. You simply lie in bed, close your eyes and imagine yourself in a calm, safe, pleasant place – the classic desert island is fine, but if you prefer, you can 'be' somewhere more meaningful to you – a bluebell wood, a favourite country spot, a cosy place in your childhood home. Move through this relaxing 'land-scape'; see if you can go into detail, using all your senses. What can you see in your relaxing place? What can you smell? Hear? Feel? Taste? Touch? Visualisation puts your brain into a calming 'zone' and this releases deep physical tension too.

How to prepare for sleep

In *Girls Own Paper*, 1888/9, Medicus suggested that 'A bottle of Vichy or Soda Water and one little dry biscuit before going to bed are often productive of a good night's sleep.' There are several modern ways to prepare for sleep that may work even better than this:

Wind-down time

You probably already know what activities wind you up (catching up on work; doing the accounts; surfing the Internet for bargains; playing online games; arguing with your teenager/spouse/neighbour). Make it your rule to avoid these stimulating activities in the hour before bed. The trick is to replace these 'wind-up' activities with 'wind-down' ones. Exhausted parents spend hours bathing, reading to and tucking up a toddler for a reason. A restful bedtime routine signals that, physically and psychologically, it's all over. It's time to settle down and (please?) sleep. As adults we sometimes need to get back to this routine: to shift gears and prepare for sleep.

For about one hour before you go to bed, institute 'wind-down time'. Do this every day. An hour of wind-down time is great, but even if you get back late from a night out, take five or ten minutes of wind-down time.

Wind-down ideas Watch a (light and undemanding) movie or TV programme; listen to calming music; have a warm bath; read a magazine; drink herbal tea or warm milk; use a foot spa/back massage cushion – or do anything else that you know will wind you down.

⟋When my doctor told me to have a warm bath each night before bed I thought he wasn't taking my sleep problems seriously. But then he explained circadian patterns – how our bodies are programmed to go to sleep when it is dark and wake up when it's light, but modern life and the electric light has stopped us from being so linked to this pattern. He then told me that a drop in body temperature encourages circadian sleep. When you get out of a warm bath, not only are your muscles and mind more relaxed, but your temperature drops: a kick-start to sleep. It works brilliantly for me. ⟍

Andy, 37, had a car accident

Things to avoid

If you've had a hard day, you may take refuge in a large meal, alcohol, and/or chocolate before you turn in. This probably seems like a good way to relax – and in the short term it might be – but, sadly, food and drink don't encourage good sleep.

- Booze: alcohol is a sleep thief. It can make you drop off fast enough, but it also has what is known as 'the rebound effect' – once it has travelled through your system you wake up, often suddenly, sometimes unpleasantly. You may then stay awake. Swap the nightcap for herbal tea.

- Caffeine: You may well already be avoiding coffee at night. But caffeine can stay in your system for a long time, so try avoiding caffeine any time after lunch. Caffeine (albeit in lower doses) crops up in other drinks and foods too: in tea, energy drinks, colas, decaffeinated tea and coffee, and – sadly – in chocolate.

- Large meals: giving your body hard work to do (that is, lots of food to digest) shortly before sleep, is the same as giving your brain a really hard and urgent problem to solve as you climb into your pyjamas – it keeps you awake.

- Exercise: vigorous physical exercise (except sex, which has miraculously sleep-inducing effects on most people) can also disrupt sleep. Avoid vigorous exercise for at least 2–3 hours before bedtime.

Adopt healthy sleep habits: make your bed a sleep zone

Good sleepers associate bed with sleep. Poor sleepers associate bed with all sorts of other activities – watching TV, working, eating, drinking, lying awake fretting. Depending on what happened to you, you may already have spent quite a lot of time in bed either at hospital or at home, or both. Bed is suddenly not just a place to sleep – it's a place to live. You may still be associating bed with a hospital-induced sense of imprisonment or helplessness. There can be other unpleasant bed associations, too, after a health crisis: pain, immobility, confusion, nausea, fear. Bed becomes a war zone in which you worry and fret, feel lonely, frustrated and scared. You need to free your bed of these associations so that it becomes a calm, restful place again.

How to make your bed a happy place:

Get out of bed

Your bed should be used for two things and only two things – sleep and sex (sex encourages sleep, so it's one activity that is allowed in bed). Think, for a moment, what you actually use your bed for. You might sit or lie in it at night (or during the day) doing things other than sleeping – reading, catching up on emails, watching TV, chatting. The advice is simple: stop. You don't need to withdraw from your bedroom completely. But you need to get off the bed itself when you want to do anything other than sleep (or have sex).

Try this instead: a calm chair

Put a squashy chair – or even a sofa if you have space – next to your bed. Sit in this 'calm chair' wrapped up warm and cosy in a dressing gown or blanket to watch the TV, read or have a quiet chat. Only get into the bed itself when you feel ready to sleep.

Use your calm chair before you get into bed at night, but also when you wake up in the night and can't get back to sleep. The idea is to reduce or even completely stop lying wide-awake and fretting in bed. When you wake in the middle of the night, give yourself 10 minutes or so to get back off to sleep. If you can't, then get out of bed and into the calm chair. Make sure that close to hand you have a blanket, a magazine or book that is not too taxing (although when it comes to 'pretty stories of love and murder' you can be your own judge), an iPod or the radio (only listen to soothing things, though). You can even go as far as having a thermos of chamomile tea by your calm chair. Only get back in bed when you feel yourself getting sleepy. If you can't sleep in bed after about 10 more minutes, get back into the calm chair and repeat until you do sleep – and you will.

HAVING DOUBTS?

As you have been reading, you've probably had your doubts about these suggestions. Thoughts like: 'This is far too complicated', 'I can't fit a chair in my room', 'My partner's lying next to me – this is going to drive her mad', 'It's far too painful for me to get in and out of bed', and so on.

Changing habits is difficult. Changing night-time habits, when you are probably at a low ebb anyway, is even harder. None of the advice, here, is set in stone. Just pick bits that work for you, and ignore others. If it's too painful or complicated to get in and out of bed into a calm chair, you could get into a different position – maybe sitting upright, or changing your pillows, or turning a night light on. This will make your 'awake' bed as different as possible from your 'sleeping' bed. If you can't fit a chair into your room, you could set up your calm chair in a next-door room. If you think, 'Fine, but I can't keep going at this for several months', then set yourself a time limit. Tell yourself you'll try these strategies for a month, then see where you've got to. You can always try the strategies for another month at some future date. The point is just to use the essence of these strategies. Don't just give up and think, 'This'll never work for me.' These are scientifically tested strategies devised by sleep experts so give them your best shot.

Partners and sleep problems

If you have a partner, the chances are you're not the only one who is fed up to the back teeth with your sleep issues. It is always worth telling your partner what your strategy is (they could read this chapter!). It might also be helpful for your partner to sleep in a spare bed while you sort out your sleep issues – just as a temporary measure. Separate rooms is a very loaded notion. And it can be hard to ask a loved-one to change their own sleep routine. It's very tempting to mind-read ('He's going to hate moving into a different room', 'She's done enough for me already, she's never going to agree to this', 'She'll think I'm rejecting her'). But temporarily moving into different rooms, far from being a sign of distance or failure, can be a constructive, relationship-strengthening solution. You can jointly decide on how long you will do this for, and set a definite end point. This is not a sign of something 'deeper' about the two of you. It's a pragmatic survival strategy.

More things to try for a good night's sleep

Adjust your sleep environment

Sometimes really simple changes to your bed and bedroom make a big difference. Think about:

- Room temperature: too much warmth can interfere with sleep, so try turning the thermostat down by two or three degrees to see if that helps.

- Uncomfortable mattress: mattresses are expensive, but they do eventually wear out. If you are still sleeping on one you bought 20 years ago, it may be time to change. If you can't afford a new mattress, a slightly cheaper option is to buy a memory foam mattress topper or the best quality mattress pad you can find.

- Outside noise: you can't control it, but earplugs may help.
- Bedroom light: darkness is good. Blackout blinds or curtains lined with blackout material are ideal, but if this is all sounding too expensive, a sleep mask or even a blanket tacked over the window can help.
- Different pillows/supports: it may be that your body now needs different pillow support. Experiment!

❝I had to sleep upright after heart surgery. It was OK in hospital because the bed was positioned correctly, but when I got home I could not get enough pillows in the right place to support me. A friend gave me a foam wedge that made all the difference.❞

Stanley, 66, had aortic valve replacement surgery

Banish lie ins

If you've slept badly, it's tempting to have a lie in, but the longer you sleep in the morning the more likely you are not to feel tired at your usual bedtime the next night. This slowly shifts your body clock – which is the opposite of what you're trying to do. Set yourself a wake-up time and stick to it – however badly you've slept.

Don't delay bedtimes

You may hold off going to bed, waiting and hoping that you'll get really tired. You eventually struggle exhausted to bed, but when your head hits the pillow your mind and body kick back into gear. The next night you stay up even later trying to avoid this – and before you know it your sleep pattern is haywire. Set a reasonable bedtime and stick to it, seven nights a week (don't change, even at weekends – be rigid).

Set yourself a sleep target

If you aren't sure what a 'reasonable' bedtime is, think about setting a sleep target. This is a target for the number of hours you are going to try to sleep. Stick to your target, even if some days you could sleep for longer (and some days you can't seem to sleep at all). A sleep target is about training your body and mind that these hours are for sleep. Your sleep target should be no fewer than five hours and no more than eight. If, for example, you decide to set a goal of six hours to start with, you might set midnight as your bedtime and six as your get-up time. Stick to this until it feels doable – you may not be solidly asleep for those six hours; you may have to get into your calm chair during the night, but you aren't feeling stressed or panicked by the six hours.

Once you have managed to sleep pretty well through that six hours (you might still have one or two waking moments, but you'll fall back to sleep fairly quickly), you could extend your sleep goal by 15 minutes at each end. Bedtime becomes 11.45 pm; get-up time is 6.15 am. Again, once you're sleeping well during those hours, if you still aren't feeling fully rested during the day, you could extend by another 15 minutes at each end. Bedtime is 11.30 pm, get-up time is 6.30 am. There is no 'eight hours' magic bullet here. The only thing that matters is that you feel rested during the day.

To nap or not to nap?

The standard advice for people with disrupted sleep is to avoid daytime naps and to restrict sleep to night times only. But if your body is still healing, and/or you are coping with fatigue, a brief daytime nap may be just what the doctor ordered (sometimes literally). Daytime naps only really become an issue if you are several weeks into your recovery and you are struggling to sleep at night. (For more about naps, see Chapter 6, page 163.)

SLEEPING PILLS – YES OR NO?

Sleeping pills can be a good quick fix. The reason we aren't all on them all the time is that the longer you use them the less effective they become, so you have to increase the dosage to get the same result. Also, some people become psychologically dependent on them.

If you do use them, it is recommended you only do so in short bursts – for 7–14 nights. The strategies in this chapter take time and perseverance, and the temptation to just go to the doctor for drugs can be overwhelming. But try to give yourself a month or so using the strategies in this chapter and not taking sleeping pills. Don't do this half-heartedly – really try. It's not a disaster if you do end up getting sleeping pills. Sometimes just knowing that you have a pill that you could take is enough to keep you calm (and that'll work in your favour).

❝Sleep disruption has been one of the worst consequences of my illness, but I don't worry like I used to. I now know that I may have an hour or so of extra reading during the night, so I always try to have a good book on the go. I've also found my calm chair helpful – things don't seem so bleak if you can sit in a comfy chair rather than lying in bed fretting. I've also been surprised that I can function fine even after a bad night. I've realised that the worry about sleep is worse than the physical lack of sleep. And now I've conquered the worry.❞

Maeve, 53, had peritonitis

*   *   *   *   *

Sleep problems really can feel overwhelming. They can affect so many aspects of life – far beyond the nights they disrupt. They can make the world seem bleak and lonely. But the strategies in this chapter really can make a vast difference. Don't expect miracles or instant results from any of this. It will take time. Some strategies will work for you, some won't. But if you persist, you will cope well with whatever the night throws at you. And this will make you feel a lot better.

NOTES FOR CARERS

'Everything that you do in a patient's room after he has "put up" for the night, increases tenfold the risk of his having a bad night. But, if you rouse him after he has fallen asleep, you do not risk, you secure him, a bad night.'

Florence Nightingale, *Notes on Nursing*, **1859**

The perils of night-time disturbance actually work this way for you too. If you are caring for someone who suffers from sleep disruption, the chances are that your sleep will be disrupted too (particularly if you share a bed, or are needed when they are awake). This sleep deprivation can be a major source of distress for everyone concerned. Here are some ways to manage it:

1 **Consider practical ways to minimise your own sleep disruption** How much do you really need to be up with them during the night? Can they manage alone? Are there practical things you can do to make this easier for them? If things are very intense, is there any possibility of respite care for a night a week so that you can guarantee some sleep? Can you find time for a power nap during the day? Carving out time to sleep is not selfish – it's essential. You will be in a better frame of mind to support them during the day if you have had a good night's sleep.

2 **Temporarily have separate rooms** If you are caring for your partner, you may now have different night-time needs – room temperature, bedclothes, trips to the bathroom, lights. There is no rule that says you have to sleep in the same room – indeed it was normal for (wealthy) Victorians to have separate rooms. It can really help you both to have separate rooms while the sleep problem is tackled (see page 193).

3 **Have wind-down time before bed** Do this yourself too. Caring for someone can be stressful, exhausting, frustrating. You will sleep better, too, if you wind down and lose the tension before bed.

4 **Encourage a set bedtime and getting-up time** This is a particularly valuable sleep strategy, and something you may have some influence over. (See page 194 for an explanation of why it's important.)

❝Richard had his heart attack at night, so when he got home sleeping was difficult. He wanted to talk, he wanted the light on, he kept the radio going all night. Eventually it became too much for both of us. He agreed to turning the light out and not talking after midnight, and I found a relaxation app that he could listen to on his iPod without disturbing me. He ended up using several different ones in the course of each night and it did gradually improve things until now he sleeps through most nights.❞

Francesca, 49, wife of Richard, 60,
who had a heart attack

EIGHT

INTIMATE RELATIONS

REBUILDING SEXUAL RELATIONSHIPS

'At some stage in normal convalescence, the patient may be troubled with an increasing gonad irritability which clearly indicates the return of a reserve of vitality.'

Dr John Bryant, *Convalescence*, 1927

'Gonad irritability' aside, sexual relationships can indeed become a minefield when you've had health problems. When you are lying in hospital, strapped up to machines and monitors, sex is undoubtedly the last thing on your mind. But as you start to feel a little better, you may realise that your relationship has been put under some strain and that things are not as they were. A health crisis can shift the balance in any intimate relationship. You may be facing new, perhaps painful or alarming, physical and emotional issues. Your roles may have changed. You may be under huge pressures – financial, practical and emotional.

It doesn't help that many of us baulk at the idea of talking about relationships and sex, and that the notion of talking to a doctor or any other medical person about sexual difficulties can feel completely outlandish. This can leave you feeling isolated, confused and distinctly gloomy about your sex life. This chapter will help you to negotiate that minefield so that you can move on – ideally with some enjoyment.

Relationship changes

There are many possible changes to a close relationship after ill health, but probably the most common are:

Physical care Often the onus of care lands firmly on your partner.

> 6 My vision and mobility were very badly damaged by my stroke. My wife has to help me wash, get to the bathroom, and eat. I feel like a terrible burden. 9
>
> **Ahmed, 77, had a stroke**

Rehabilitation You may have to get to grips with medication, exercises, diets and appointments, and those close to you can feel the pressure too.

> 6 My wife takes time off work to come to my physiotherapy appointments and takes on a lot of responsibility. I think she sees herself as my personal physiotherapist, although I prefer to call her my physio terrorist. 9
>
> **Darren, 47, had spinal surgery**

Changed roles These may be obvious (for example, an adult child caring for an elderly or frail parent or a change in the family breadwinner). But there can be more subtle changes too. If the person who does the driving or cooking, or the school run or the finances, has changed, feathers can be ruffled.

> 6 My partner got much more involved with the children while I was going through treatment and he found he

really liked it. But as I got better it became more complicated – we couldn't both make their packed lunches and take them to school. I felt I'd been pushed aside.

Monique, 35, had breast cancer

Money worries This is a huge one. It can affect relationships profoundly, causing great stress, unhappiness and tension.

I can't work, and I have had to go on sickness benefits, and my wife has given up her job to care for me. It feels like a double whammy. First the health went, then the money.

Tony, 57, had a heart attack

Loneliness Others assume you're through the 'eye of the storm' so you're going to pick up where you left off. If you feel this isn't happening you can feel very alone.

I look OK, I sound OK. My husband wants me to be OK, but I've actually never felt more vulnerable. I feel disconnected from him – he just doesn't get it.

Abigail, 33, had a TIA (mini stroke)

Guilt You might feel you've wrecked things (plans, lifestyle, finances). You've put others through 'so much'. You may feel like a 'burden'. Your partner, meanwhile, might feel guilty for carrying on, for being fit, for not being able to heal you, for resenting your illness.

I find the worst moment of my day is shutting the door and going off to work when Ade is at home. I know he is going to be alone for the day and it breaks my heart.

Veronica, wife of Adeola, 49, who is on kidney dialysis

Anger This is a natural response to loss and distress. You may direct this anger at a loved one, or at yourself – or both. Your partner may be bottling up anger too – life has changed, everything feels more complex.

> ❝I thought that Mike would look after me during my recovery, but he was useless. He went out more, he complained more, and in the end I moved back in with my mum. I was so furious with Mike I could barely look at him.❞
>
> **Dee, 39, had abdominal surgery**

Protectiveness Sometimes you want to protect each other from 'difficult' feelings, so you don't talk about them. Again, this can bring great tensions, loneliness and misunderstandings.

> ❝I'd lie awake at night, frightened to close my eyes in case I never woke up again. But I wouldn't wake my husband up, he needed his sleep and I didn't want to worry him.❞
>
> **Dilys, 74, had a heart attack**

Opening up the cracks Sometimes, a health crisis turns the cracks in a relationship into gaping chasms.

> ❝There were problems in our marriage before the stroke, but we'd papered them over, filling the gaps with a very busy life. The stroke finished us off. My wife became the sole breadwinner and was under enormous stress. Our plans to retire to France evaporated. Communication was zero. She shouted all the time and I withdrew. It was unsustainable.❞
>
> **Charles, 67, had a stroke**

How to manage conflict

Many of these relationship strains lead to one thing: conflict. There is a media image that after an argument couples leap into bed for a passionate resolution, but in reality conflict often does the opposite – it prevents intimacy.

Finding ways to resolve or handle conflict are essential if you are to get past this difficult time in your relationship. Here are some key conflict-resolution skills to try:

- Use 'I' messages rather than 'you'; for example, 'I don't like it when you go to the pub after work' rather than 'You always go to the pub after work!' 'I' messages make the other person feel less attacked and will bring defences down a bit.

- Stay focused on the immediate issue. Don't drag up resentments from ancient arguments that have run their course, or start saying 'and another thing . . . '

- Repeat your point: possibly several times, perhaps in different ways – calmly. Accept that sometimes this is necessary and it isn't a sign that the other person doesn't care or isn't listening.

- Aim for compromise, not victory. A balanced solution tends to be better for relationships than a win–lose outcome – even if you have to let some things go.

- Move on. Going back over a disagreement keeps the topic 'hot' and stores up future resentment.

- Don't sulk – if you are still bothered, address the issue directly. Other people aren't mind-readers, even if you think they should be. They may have no idea why you are sulking and cross. All sulking does is prolong the agony.

TIP

Get help

If you've reached a point where conflicts are overwhelming, and none of these conflict-resolution strategies seems to work, help from a professional third party can be invaluable. If your boiler breaks and your central-heating system collapses, you aren't going to soldier on through the winter thinking, 'it might get better'. You'll call an engineer to diagnose and solve the problem. There is no shame in getting relationship help – and it is not a sign that things are 'dire' or 'unfixable'. Organisations such as Relate are well aware of the massive strains that ill health can put on relationships.

Sexual hurdles

These are less energetic than they sound, but it is worth thinking about this to work out what's really going on if your sex life seems complicated or non-existent. Common sexual problems after a health crisis include:

Fear and worry Fear that sex will provoke a heart attack or stroke, dislocate a newly positioned hip, split a wound or disrupt any other healing process is not sexy. Add in worries about pain during sex (either causing it or feeling it), as well as that old favourite, performance anxiety, and sex can quickly seem out of the question.

> ❛Having sex for the first time after my heart attack was one of the scariest things I have ever done. I was convinced that the increase in blood pressure and heart

rate would trigger another attack. But of course I was fine, and with time the fear has gone, but it did take a very long time.⁹

Douglas, 62, had a heart attack

Loss of confidence When your body has been battered, bruised or cut, it is not easy to feel confident. The loss of body parts or functions, the addition of scars or weight, pain or difficulty with movement can all make you feel profoundly unconfident in bed. This may get better with time, but often you do have to tackle this lack of confidence, and build it back up again, before sex can seem possible.

⁶I feel different, less attractive and less sexual now. I know it sounds silly but I used to love getting dressed up for a night out, putting on a sexy dress, high heels and so on, but since I've put on weight and the pain in my leg means I can only wear big clumpy flat shoes, I just don't make the effort. I don't believe that my partner can still find me attractive. I feel unattractive and I just don't want to try making love.⁹

Lesley, 46, broke her pelvis in a car crash

Depression Low mood and depression can affect your libido. Depressed thoughts such as 'I am unattractive', 'I am worthless', 'I am unlovable' are a huge barrier to intimate relationships.

⁶I can't imagine who would want to have a relationship with me – a man full of cancer and chemotherapy, feeling sorry for himself. I'm hardly a very good catch.⁹

Solomon, 39, had kidney cancer

Sexual function Ill health and its treatments can directly affect sexual functions such as the ability to get and maintain an erection, vaginal lubrication, arousal, orgasm or, more generally, libido. Pain, numbness or movement difficulties can also reduce sexual desire or pleasure. These can be huge hurdles.

❝I am numb on my left side now, so sex feels different. It is OK and sometimes I do enjoy it, but at other times I find it a bit upsetting as it reminds me of the loss of feeling in my left side.❞

Jane, 57, had a stroke

All of these hurdles can be tackled and improved, if you know how.

'Gonad irritability': is it dangerous?

What if, by having sex, you do yourself an injury, set back your progress, or do really serious damage? Scenes on TV or in movies where people clutch at their chest and keel over during sex are pretty much a media staple. You could be forgiven for thinking that all you have to do is think about sex and it's curtains. This is a particularly vivid worry if you have had a heart attack or a stroke, but, in fact, this sort of fear is not based on any kind of medical accuracy. The reality is that, despite what the television dramas would have us believe, fewer than 1 per cent of heart attacks or strokes occur during sex. Indeed, of the few that do happen during sex, most may not have been triggered by the sex itself: those heart attacks were going to happen anyway.

As long as you follow your doctor's recommendations, and do not simply spring from the hospital trolley straight into your love nest, sex will do you no harm. In fact – if your doctor has OK'd it – sex is likely to make you feel a lot better!

COMMON MYTHS ABOUT SEX AFTER A HEALTH CRISIS

MYTH Sex after heart attack/stroke/cancer/surgery is dangerous.

REALITY Sex is safe, and could enhance well-being and recovery. Always check with your doctor first, but in the vast majority of cases, sex after a health crisis is not just harmless, it's positively good for you.

MYTH It is not appropriate to use up a doctor's time talking about sexual problems.

REALITY Most people involved in your health care will want to help you and will be experienced in talking about sex after illness or injury. It may feel awkward to raise the issue, and they may (like you) struggle to start the conversation for fear of embarrassing you, or seeming intrusive, but health professionals can be a brilliant source of expert advice, medical reassurance and information.

MYTH It is not possible to have sex if you have weakness/pain/disability.

REALITY You'll probably have to make some adjustments when it comes to planning, positioning and pace, but sex is both possible and enjoyable, even when you are dealing with all sorts of physical challenges.

MYTH Penetrative sex is the only sex worth having.

REALITY This rules out a lot. Think back over your sexual history. There will probably be episodes of great sex that did not involve penetration. We have, in fact, become a bit hung up on the idea that only penetrative sex counts. Depending on your recovery issues it is possible that non-penetrative sex might be your best bet.

MYTH If you have sexual problems, you just have to live with them.

REALITY There are loads of things that can be done to get your sex life back on track after a serious illness or injury. There is no need to give up or suffer in silence.

Waiting until you're 'ready'

You may hear or read (probably online) that you should 'wait until you feel ready' before you have sex again. This is all well and good, but it completely ignores the fear factor. If you have not spoken directly to your doctor about re-starting your sex life, you will almost certainly have absorbed the myth that sex is going to be dangerous. This lack of information really does hold us back. Studies show that people who are given advice from their medical teams about when to start having sex again after a heart attack are more likely to be sexually active than those who get no advice. Sadly most of us don't ask.

❛I felt very adrift after my surgery, particularly when it came to making love. I looked on the Internet but couldn't find any information that seemed trustworthy. In the end I plucked up the courage to talk to a friend who'd been through a similar procedure. She reassured me that sex could still be safe and fun.❜

Nell, 61, had a hysterectomy

When it's safe to have sex will depend on your health condition and your individual needs. When it comes to sex after a heart attack or stroke, the very general medical consensus is that you should wait until you can walk comfortably up two flights of stairs without chest pain or significant breathlessness. Another common piece of advice is to wait four to six weeks after a heart attack or stroke. Six weeks is also generally the magic number when it comes to sex after surgery. But by far the best way to know for sure what's safe for you is to ask your doctor. As you turn down the lights you do not want any niggling worry standing between you and your loved one.

Sex and medications

Many medications can affect your sexual function including your libido or ability to become aroused. Medications can also be prescribed to help your sex life. Your doctor (family medical practitioner or specialist) may be able to tweak your medication to avoid these side effects, or perhaps prescribe drugs such as Viagra to help with arousal. Don't try to bypass the potential embarrassment of talking to a doctor and get pills or other treatments on the Internet – this can be anything from ineffective and expensive to downright dangerous.

TIP

Body logistics

It can help enormously to think through the logistics of having sex in advance: plan your positions, gather cushions or other supports if parts of your body are going to need propping up. If you have had surgery, you'll need to avoid positions that put pressure on the wound or scar area or put weight on a new joint. Planning sounds unsexy, but it can make a vast difference.

Your mind: overcoming mental or emotional hurdles

Your thoughts, feelings and fears can be even more of an obstacle to intimacy than your body. Here are some ways to tackle the 'mind' hurdles:

1 **Face up to fear and doubt** If you are afraid that sex may damage you in some way, your doctor is probably the only person who can really convince you that sex won't do you any harm – indeed, it may do you a lot of good.

2 **Focus on foreplay** This can allow your anxiety to settle, and everything else to kick in gradually.

3 **Monitor your physical sensations – without fear** During sex your heart will beat faster, your breathing will speed up, certain muscles will tense or tire. You know this is normal, but after a health crisis innocuous bodily sensations can take on ominous overtones. If you remind yourself (perhaps in advance) that feeling hot, breathing fast, noticing your heart beating are all normal, you won't be freaked out when these things happen. Again, your doctor can give you a list of symptoms that are not OK (depending on your health issue, this could include things like chest pain, unusual palpitations, sharp pain or dizziness). If you have this information, you won't confuse potentially great sensations with alarm bells, or spend your whole time worrying about what might be happening to your body.

4 **Beware Thought Traps** Thoughts will be crowding into your head before, during and after sex. If you are saying harsh or punishing things to yourself ('Oh no, my heart is racing, this must be dangerous', 'We'll never make love spontaneously again', 'This is going to hurt like hell'), you are unlikely to feel sexy. Your thoughts can intensify any fear or depression or lack of confidence. Try to acknowledge what you are thinking. Consider your 'case for the defence': 'I am with my loving partner', 'There have been changes and losses but we are both trying to give it a go', 'Let's just have a go – we don't need to make the earth move.' It also helps to manage your expectations about what sex will be like: it may not be perfect, but when is sex perfect, really? Afterwards, instead of focusing on what wasn't ideal, try to think about what did go right: did you look into each other's eyes? Did you talk afterwards? Did you feel close, even fleetingly?

5 **Try to laugh** If it was an unmitigated disaster – or even just a bit daft – humour can really help. Sex is sometimes a bit ridiculous, ungainly, absurd and occasionally downright dreadful. And it can be more so if you are grappling with physical restrictions and emotional hurdles. Laughter is a fantastic way to release tension, let it go, move on – together.

6 **Talk, talk, talk** There are enough opportunities for miscommunication and misunderstanding in relationships in general, but when you add health problems to the mix, the confusion can skyrocket. You might think your partner has lost interest – he may simply be afraid that he'll hurt you. You might think your partner doesn't find you attractive any more – she may be struggling with arousal because of her medication. Such scenarios (the confusions and misunderstandings are practically limitless when it comes to sex) could be avoided if only we'd *talk* to each other about our sexual needs and feelings.

Try this: sex talk

Sex talk time is not quite as thrilling as it sounds. It's all very well being told to 'talk, talk, talk' but you may need a clearer plan than that. With sex talk, you and your partner agree on a specific time (maybe a regular time during the week) where you will sit down together and talk about your sex life. Keep this short – no more than about half an hour at a time. Even 10 minutes is a great start.

A good starting point is to ask: *what, actually, do we want?*

You might, for example, assume that your partner needs to have penetrative sex, whereas they might just be desperate for the emotional closeness of lying in bed together, hugging. Finding out what you both want, and expect, can be a revelation. You can then agree a mutual goal, and talk about how to achieve it. You may find that you need help to sort out these issues – they can be emotive, complicated, hidden.

If sex talk isn't working for you, expert sexual counselling might really help. There are also online counselling organisations (see Resources), which allow you to stay anonymous, and may be useful if it is hard for you to get to appointments.

How to talk to health professionals about sex

So you've now been badgered, constantly, about talking to your doctor. But, what if talking to your doctor (or specialist nurse, or physio) about sex is an utterly mortifying prospect? Here are some strategies for tackling the very common 'cringe-factor'.

Lay good groundwork Know what you want to ask, who you want to ask and how long you think you might need. Perhaps it would be good to book a double appointment with the doctor? Think about who you are talking to. Would it be easier to talk to your specialist nurse rather than the doctor? Could you ask to speak to your consultant in private, if you walk into the consulting room and find that half the medical school are sitting there too? Would a female or male doctor be best (if there is a choice)?

Think about what – or who – to take along Write down your questions and take them with you – this can help if you can't seem to think clearly. If you have seen any leaflets that outline the kinds of difficulties you are having, you could take them and use that to kick off the conversation. Or, there may be an online resource or article you've seen that you could print out and refer to. Also, do think about whether you want to seek this advice on your own or with your partner.

What to say

Sometimes just getting the words out can feel awkward. This is going to sound mad, but it can help to practise, in advance, what you're going to say to the doctor.

1 General advice on when to resume sex: you don't need to be explicit or go into any detail. You could say, 'I'd like to know when it's safe to have sex again', 'Can you tell me when it would be safe for me to have intercourse again?', 'My partner and I were wondering whether it is safe to resume our sex life?'

2 Specific advice on a sexual issue: you could start with: 'I have some concerns about how my illness has affected my sex life. Can I talk to you about them?'

TIP

Avoid euphemisms

They'll only make you more uncomfortable. If you aren't happy using the word 'sex', try 'intercourse' or even, at a pinch, 'marital relations', but if you can, in general, it is far better to just say what you mean – clearly and succinctly.

It can be hard to use words like 'vagina' or 'penis' or 'erection', but you will find the conversation far less embarrassing if you just come out and name the body parts. These people have been to medical school. They've dealt endlessly with human bodies. You can't shock them. It can help to practise the words out loud. When you're sure you're alone, and no one is listening, try just saying it several times.

For example: 'I am finding it hard to get an erection and wondered if there are medical reasons for this, and ways to treat it.' Or 'I'm finding I have quite bad vaginal dryness and pain during intercourse since surgery, is there anything you could prescribe that might tackle this problem?'

Health professionals say these words frequently and they won't flinch when you say them – they won't even really notice. They'll just be grateful you're being clear and not talking around the subject using euphemisms.

When the sex stops completely

If your sex life has ground to a halt and none of this chapter has felt remotely meaningful to you, it's time to go back to basics. First, try to work out why your sex life has stopped. Try asking yourself these questions:

- Has my health caused physical issues that make sex seem impossible? If so, what are these, specifically?

- Are changes to our relationship causing us to feel distant? If so, what are our main relationship changes?

- Has my health caused me so much fear, shame or discomfort that I just can't face sex? If so, what are my fears specifically?

- Has my health triggered an underlying problem in my relationship, which is now illuminated even more by the lack of sex?

If you and your partner both genuinely have no desire for a sex life, that is completely fine. Plenty of couples are non-sexual, and very happy. But it is important to know for sure that this is mutual. It's no good if one person is just 'being nice' or 'trying to be supportive' by saying they don't want sex any more either, when really they're upset or saddened by the lack of sex.

If one or both of you aren't perfectly content with the lack of sex, then this is a pretty major issue, no matter how much you, or your partner, downplay it. It can really help to address this with a therapist so that it doesn't snowball into a very unhappy situation. You can find help from organisations such as Relate, online counselling or from a psychosexual doctor via The Institute of Psychosexual Medicine (see Resources).

If your sex life has stalled and you both know you want to get it going again, here are some tried-and-tested strategies:

Try this: go slowly

Start by *not* having sex. Yes, OK, you're already not having sex, but you are probably feeling a huge pressure to have sex, and thinking that if only you could force yourself in some way, then you would have sex. This sort of pressure often leads to tension and worry. Instead, try to rebuild your physical closeness brick by brick without the pressure of a 'goal' (penetrative sex).

The idea is to only go back to full sexual intercourse when you have worked through the steps below and you both decide that this is what you want. For some couples, this may take a few weeks, but for others it may be months. There is no 'set time'.

Instead of having sex:

- Build emotional intimacy. Spend some time each day talking and listening to each other, touching, showing affection, making eye contact, cuddling, kissing (but no penetrative sex).

- Hold hands or touch when going out for a walk or while watching TV.

- After a week or fortnight of this emotional 'building' (whatever timescale you choose), move to the next step: add in some kissing (but away from the bedroom).

- After you've focused on kissing and closeness for another week or so, move to the next step: kissing in bed. Again, do this for a week or so – or longer. But no sex. Even if you feel you might like it. Removing the option of sex is liberating. It stops one person feeling they 'should' because the other clearly wants to. It's a rule: no sex.

- When you're ready, add in hugging, touching and foreplay – in stages. Still no penetrative sex. Be really firm on that. You have to keep the pressure off.

- If you do want to go on to penetrative sex, only do so after you've done the stages above over several weeks.

Remember: penetrative sex is not everything. Your goal may be simply to feel close and connected.

TIP

Consider taking more of a back seat

When you do start having intercourse, you could talk with your partner about taking a slightly more passive role during sex than you usually do. It can feel odd to control your movements or pace, but you'll get used to it – and it might really help if you have physical restrictions. If you talk about this in advance, you won't be worrying, and it won't feel so odd for both of you.

Sex with a new partner

Of course, sex doesn't just happen in long-term, loving relationships. You may be single and thinking, perhaps with some trepidation, about your future sex life. The dating scene is hard enough when we're fully fit and raring to go, but it can be a whole lot harder when you add in health issues.

❝I had been divorced for five years before I had my heart surgery. I convinced myself that the sex side of my life was over and I felt OK about it. Then I met a really lovely man in the Tesco car park! He saw me struggling with my shopping, helped me and then asked me out. We have taken things very slowly, but regaining a sex life that I thought was over has been a lovely surprise for me, especially at my age.❞

Joy, 68, had heart bypass surgery

Whatever your situation, try to think in advance how you're going to handle any of the physical hurdles you may now be dealing with.

Prepare your 'line' If you have an obvious physical restriction or scar or disability, it can help to prepare what you'll say about this to a new (or potential) partner. Anything that feels right to you is fine, but think about how much detail you want to go into. Anything from 'I have a few battle scars', or 'The years have rather taken their toll', to a clear explanation about what has happened to you and how this affects your performance is fine. It's up to you. Again, gentle humour in this situation can be helpful, if it feels right.

Think ahead If you have an inkling that you might become more serious about this person, you could consider talking to them about what you've been through before you become sexually intimate. There are risks here because of the other person's fear, or their own issues (maybe they have had a brush with health problems too), or sometimes people just turn out not to be very nice. But the ones who stick around will be there because they really want to be with you – warts (OK, cancer, heart attack, stroke, surgical scars, and so on) and all.

Consider when to talk Your health and recovery is, of course, a major part of who you are, but it doesn't define you, any more than your family background, relationship history or job does. Trust your instinct on when to talk. It might take several conversations with a new or potential sexual partner to introduce your health history, and a lot more before you are ready for a more detailed conversation about scars, lubrication, positioning, erectile function and so on.

❝I thought I'd never find anyone who'd want to be with me, but it turns out I was wrong. I broke up with my fiancée soon after my cancer – not because of the cancer, but because we just weren't right for each other. The stress of my illness demonstrated that to us, loud and clear. Then I met my wife. She was scared by my health history, but we talked a lot, and about my disability, and that brought us much closer, much faster – and the closeness enhanced our sex life!❞

Frank, 38, who had colon cancer, and has a stoma

* * * * *

The relationship between sex and illness has always been complex. In the 19th century, tuberculosis was seen by some as a 'disease of passion' – the fever was a sign of 'an inward burning', the disease was the 'ravages of frustration' and the patient was undoubtedly 'consumed by ardour'. Indeed, sex was also prescribed as a treatment for tuberculosis. In Henry James's novel, *The Wings of the Dove*, Milly Theale is advised to have a love affair to cure her TB. Fortunately, we have moved away from such bonkers ideas, but when it comes to sex as a healing force for good, there could be something to it.

Right now, your sex life (or lack of it?) may feel anything but healing or life enhancing. It may feel like a final straw, a lost cause, or another stress to face. Your intimate relationship may not be exactly what it was. It may take very unsexy amounts of time, planning, self-examination, effort and talking to get there. But you will get there in the end, so don't lose hope. Give some of these strategies a try. You'll be surprised at how effective they can be.

NOTES FOR CARERS

If you are caring for your partner, the chances are that your sex life has been affected in some way – probably not for the best. This chapter has explained why this can happen, so if you haven't read it – please do. The information and advice here also applies to you. After you've read the chapter, try to:

1 **Talk about it with your partner** Did any of it ring true for you? Which strategies did you find helpful? Were there any things you disagree with? Talking will help you to narrow down (if you don't know already) what your main concerns are. Now, you can decide, together, what you'd like to work on, using the ideas in the chapter.

2 **Knock fear on the head** If you are afraid to have sex, try to identify what, exactly, you are afraid of. Often the partner of someone who has had health problems will be afraid of causing physical pain or harm, or of being too demanding. See if you can talk to your partner about your fears. It may also be a good idea to talk to someone from the health care team – even though this can be hard to contemplate. (See pages 212–13 on how to talk to health professionals about sex.) If you stay silent, it's easy for confusion, misunderstanding and hurt to take hold, and this can damage any relationship.

3 **Try to accept the changes** Try to talk about the changes together. You may even need to acknowledge that they are permanent. If this is hard for you, it's OK to say so. Your partner may be feeling something similar, with extra guilt added on top. The only way to understand each other and move on is to be honest.

4 **Seek professional help** Don't let shyness, embarrassment or shame hold you back from talking to a sexual or relationships

therapist. They certainly aren't going to be embarrassed, so why should you be? Getting help from someone who specialises in relationships could be the key to recovering both your emotional and physical intimacy.

6Evelyn and I got into a terrible muddle about sex after her breast cancer surgery. I was afraid of hurting her and was waiting for her to signal to me when she felt ready. She, meanwhile, was thinking that I couldn't look at her scars and didn't find her attractive any more. We lived in a world of silence and hurt. This was only relieved when she went for counselling and the therapist asked me to come into a couple of the sessions as well.9

Robert, 50, husband of Evelyn, 48, who had breast cancer

NINE

THE STUFFING PROCESS

STRATEGIES FOR EATING WELL

In 1904, *Fannie Farmer's Food and Cookery for the Sick and Convalescent* outlined a treatment for the consumptive, which included a high and dry climate, a liberal supply of fresh cold air, a cold-water bath each morning, light physical exercise, and a 'stuffing process'. During this 'stuffing process' the convalescent was offered plenty of 'easily digested food' including eggs, cream, butter, olive oil, bacon and beef fat. Doctors at that time particularly recommended eggs – as many as 18 a day, but Farmer did not approve of such excess: 'Patients', she wrote, 'usually tire of eggs when taken in such large numbers.' Her top tip for settling the stomach after an ill-advised egg binge? An alcoholic drink.

Nowadays, top doctors don't tend to recommend 18 eggs and a dram to those who want to feel better. But if you ignore your diet, or assume it doesn't matter, you are missing a trick. Eating healthily should be a basic element of your recovery plan – whatever has happened to you.

Exactly what or how much you should eat will depend on many factors – from your appetite to your mobility, bodily needs, personal taste and, of course, your particular health condition. Sadly, this book cannot offer you a bespoke diet plan, but there are some common dietary concerns faced by people with health problems, and if you know how to negotiate them, you will be able to eat sensibly, and well. Doing so can make a huge difference to how you feel.

COMMON OBSTACLES TO HEALTHY EATING
AFTER ILLNESS OR INJURY:

1 Working out what's best to eat for your particular health
condition.

2 Making the dietary changes recommended by your
medical team.

3 Coping with loss of appetite or appetite/taste changes.

4 Coping with the practicalities of food shopping and
preparation – mobility issues, fatigue.

5 Building yourself up after hospitalisation – tackling
weight loss and general lack of vitality.

What is healthy eating?

Probably the biggest favour you can do yourself is to learn
about the basics of healthy eating. You may already have
absorbed some of the most important public health messages
about eating well (see box opposite). But let's get realistic here.
It can be hard enough to put healthy-eating advice into practice
when you're fit and well. But when you are dealing with very
specific challenges – emotional, physical or practical – eating
well gets even harder.

If, for example, you are malnourished after hospitalisation (and
many people are), how do you build yourself back up? If you are
living alone and have mobility problems, how do you shop for
and prepare a healthy meal? If you've just recovered from a serious illness, how do you choose foods that will give you energy
and strength? And how do you know what eating advice in the
media is good and what's nonsense – should you be guzzling goji
berries? Quaffing spirulina shakes? Cutting out whole food
groups? Blowing your life savings on vitamin supplements?

HEALTHY EATING: THE BASICS

In essence, this is what you need to know about eating a balanced diet:

- Eat at least five portions of fruit and vegetables every day. Fruit and vegetables are best for your 'five-a-day', but one glass of fruit juice to replace one of those portions is also fine, particularly if you are struggling to eat enough fruit and vegetables. Try to make your plate a 'rainbow'; that is, include different colours of fruits and vegetables with every meal (such as, broccoli, sweetcorn, a red pepper and an orange).

- Drink plenty of fluids – we need at least 1.2 litres (2 pints) of fluid a day (about eight glasses). Water is ideal.

- Include at least two portions of fish in your diet per week, aim for one or two portions of oily fish (oily fish includes salmon, mackerel or sardines and contains omega-3 fats, which may protect you against heart disease).

- Opt for whole grains and wholewheat, when it comes to starches like bread, pasta or rice. Switch to brown rice, wholewheat pasta, and choose breads such as a wholemeal loaf or Granary. These are great sources of dietary fibre and contain more nutrients than white starches.

- Eat only very small amounts of saturated fats – make cakes, biscuits, crisps and chips only an occasional treat. Use butter and dairy produce in moderation.

- Include some 'good fats' in your diet. These are found in foods such as olive oil, avocado, plain nuts or seeds, such as sunflower seeds, pumpkin seeds or sesame seeds – try sprinkling them on salads or in soups.

This really is just the bare bones, but for more information and more detailed explanations see Resources.

Why bother?

Studies show that good nutrition improves disease recovery, with fewer complications and shorter hospital stays. Poor nutrition, on the other hand, can cause muscle wasting and weakness, decrease your mobility and stamina, impair your lung and heart functions, cause poor wound healing, impair your immune responses, delay recovery from illness and cause a higher incidence of post-operative complications. One study by the British Dietetic Association found that 40 per cent of people admitted to hospital were suffering from malnutrition. This doesn't mean they were all thin. You can be overweight and malnourished. Malnutrition is when you are either not eating enough, or not eating a wide enough range of food to meet your body's needs. In short: whatever your health issue, if you want to feel better faster it's worth focusing on what you eat.

How to get good dietary information

Specific dietary advice can be hard to find. You may end up scraping together bits and pieces of information from doctors, nurses, the media, the Internet and friends. This can lead to considerable confusion. Here are some ways to find the information you need:

Ask your health-care team for dietary advice If possible, it is better to make an appointment to discuss your dietary needs and concerns, rather than tack the conversation on to an existing appointment. If you try to tack it on, the chances are it will get lost – or squeezed into a few moments at the end and you'll come away none the wiser. Instead, say clearly that you are confused about what to eat for your health, and that you need help and guidance. You may or may not end up with all the information you need, but it is definitely your best starting point.

Consult your health charity If there is a registered health charity associated with your particular medical condition, this can be an invaluable source of reliable, evidence-based dietary information. At the very least, there might be a helpline staffed by someone who can point you in the right direction.

Ignore newspaper or magazine articles about 'superfoods' or 'miracle diets' or 'food that will save your life'. The information in these articles is almost always unreliable, partial, wildly inflated – and often just downright wrong.

Educate yourself on the solid, research-based basics It is surprising how many people think, 'Yes, yes, I know about healthy eating', but do not, in fact, understand some of the real nuts and bolts – the basic food groups or the need to reduce saturated fats or salt (and what that means when you're looking at a food label). These might seem like obvious or boring things to consider, but they will make a huge difference to your health and well-being if you put them into practice. If you understand the food groups, for example, you can look at what foods don't agree with you and swap them for another food in that group, rather than just cutting them out and eating a less balanced diet.

Avoid random websites about individual foods or eating strategies If there was overwhelming clinical evidence that one way of eating was going to provide the elixir of youth, make you live forever, and protect you against all known disease, doctors would be recommending it. Often the things you find online that seem 'informative' are by commercial companies trying to flog you foods or supplements or diet books.

> **TIP**
>
> ---
>
> **Eat like great grandma**
>
> Another useful healthy-eating rule is to only eat foods that your great grandmother would have recognised as *food*. This directs you to simple, wholesome foods – fruits, vegetables, beans, whole grains, fish and lean meats without nasty additives, added high-fructose corn syrup, artificial flavours, colours or trans-fats which are simply not good for any of us. Clearly, this won't always be possible, but wherever you can, think about great grandma.

Loss of appetite

This is very common after a range of health issues. Most people, for example, lose 5–10 per cent of their body weight after having major surgery. If you have been overweight, weight loss may seem like a blessing, but if you lose too much weight too fast, you can become undernourished. If your body is not getting the nutrition it needs, it will have to work harder to fight infection, heal injury and rebuild muscle strength. This will stop you feeling better.

❝I lost almost 2 stone while I was ill. At first I felt like it was the one good side effect of the infection, but after I'd been home for a while I started to worry, because my weight loss was making me feel weak, debilitated and tired.❞

Errol, 52, had septicaemia

Victorian doctors recommended 'good plain food' for convales-cents, and this is actually a fine place to start when thinking about appetite. Mrs Beeton sensibly said, 'For invalids, never make a large quantity of one thing, as they seldom require much at a time; and it is desirable that variety be provided for them.' Victorian beef tea, along with lambs' tongues, liver pie, pobble (sausages boiled in milk), sweetbreads, tripe, eels, oysters and calves' foot jelly may not sound terribly tempting, but it is a good idea to give some thought to making food appetising. Choose whole foods (rather than processed ones) that are simple to prepare, easy to eat and packed with nutrients. Try not to worry too much about the quantity you are eating, but do think about the quality. If you aren't able to eat much, you want to maximise the nutrients you are getting with every mouthful.

Try:

Soups If you are up to cooking (or someone is willing to cook for you) a large batch of soup that doesn't taste too strong and isn't too complicated to prepare, is a great idea. Ideally, it should include plenty of vegetables as well as some protein (such as pulses, fish, chicken, beef). This makes a nutrient-dense meal that's easy to eat (a 'meal in a bowl'). If you have the where-withal to make a batch and freeze, you have an easy supply of healthy ready meals (just freeze them in individual portions).

Smoothies You can get many of your five-a-day fruits (or vegetables) by whizzing them in a blender, when you are not feeling up to solid meals. Again, to minimise the effort, aim to whizz a great big jug and keep it in the fridge – you can take small drinks throughout the day.

Add-ins Lizzie Heritage, in her book *Cookery for Invalids and Others* (1897), suggested having a glass of champagne, if you feel sick, and adding cream to it for extra 'body'. The strategy behind this historical oddity is actually quite solid: having a snack with your cup of tea, adding calorie-dense food such as a handful of nuts or an avocado to your salad, or some extra cheese to your mashed potatoes, can help if you are trying to regain weight.

Shakes/build ups/sip feeds You can either buy these over the counter or get them on prescription from your doctor. You don't have to live on them forever, but they can be a handy addition to your kitchen cabinet for when you simply don't have the energy or ability to cook. A health professional – your doctor, a dietician, nurse or pharmacist – will be able to advise you on which are the most practical and helpful for you right now.

Make it look good Fannie Farmer wrote in 1904 that 'The trays should be of correct size, so when laid not to have the appearance of being overcrowded ... The tray cloth should be spotless and just fit over the edge of the tray. Select the choicest china, silver and glasswear ... make the breakfast tray as attractive as possible by using bright flowers.' The modern-day equivalent of this fussing is simply to think about what might appeal to you most; a small portion can seem more manageable than a pile of food, for example. Food served on a nice plate really can look more appealing than in the packet (that's why posh restaurants use those huge white plates with drizzles and garnishes). Appetite is not just about taste, it's about sensation – sight, smell, texture.

Superfoods: should I be eating them?

Celery, broccoli, jam, popcorn and cereals have all been hyped as superfoods in the past few years. We've also been told that anything, from garlic to chocolate, to – yes really – two and a half bottles of wine a week, can 'save your life'. Media claims for individual foods (or drinks) are almost always wildly exaggerated – and often just plain wrong. A newspaper article that said, 'nobody really knows whether chocolate is good or bad for you' or 'lots more studies are needed to establish whether green tea protects against prostate cancer' would not generate many Twitter comments or sell glossy magazines. There is actually no such thing as a 'superfood'. The evidence-based route to good nutrition is to eat a balanced and varied diet – including a range of foods. If you do this, and limit your intake of alcohol and high-fat, high-sugar, salty and processed foods, quit smoking, try to keep to a healthy weight and take part in regular physical activity you will see far more progress than if you eat a head of garlic a day or blow your life savings on a bunch of kukicha twigs.

TIP

Drink more fluids

If you aren't able to eat well, it is easy to get dehydrated. Water makes up around 70 per cent of the human body – it's important for digestion, joint function, healthy skin and removal of waste products. Sometimes fatigue, lightheadedness or nausea can be caused by dehydration (you can also tell if you're dehydrated if your urine is dark and strong smelling).

As stated earlier, you should be aiming to drink around 1.2 litres (2 pints) of fluids a day. You may feel quite different (more energetic and alert) if you do manage this. If you are worried about constantly going to the loo, or if drinking is difficult, try sipping very small amounts throughout the day (roughly eight glasses of water a day in total). It doesn't have to be only plain water: diluted fruit juices or herbal teas all are fine if you need a change from plain water. Bear in mind that the caffeine in coffee and tea, and some fizzy drinks, will make you want to go to the loo even more often.

Food supplements – yes or no?

Even though we spend millions every year on dietary supplements, the scientific evidence about vitamin and mineral supplements is inconclusive. The current advice is therefore to get your daily vitamins and minerals from a variety of real food. If you do decide to take a vitamin supplement, make sure to mention it to your doctor, but don't fall into the trap of thinking, 'It doesn't matter what I eat because I took my multivitamin pill.'

Coping with dietary changes

Whether you have been told you have high cholesterol, are at risk of diabetes, need to lose weight or have to follow any other new regime, changing eating habits can feel difficult, depressing and confusing.

Your toolkit for success

1 **Get personalised advice** The quality and quantity of information we get when we have to make dietary changes varies massively. One person might be handed a very basic leaflet, whereas another might be offered expert, individual advice, support and follow-up. A general healthy-eating booklet is not specific enough: you need advice that's tailored to you and your personal health issue. The best place to start is by asking your medical team. There may be nurses with expertise, or even nutritional advisors, who can talk you through practical ways to make changes. Your doctor may be able to refer you to a dietician. Go on the principle of 'don't ask, don't get'; you may end up with nothing, or you may get the help and support you need. It's worth a try.

2 **Set smaller, realistic goals for yourself** The ideal goal is SMART: Specific, Measurable, Achievable, Realistic and Timely (see page 115). Instead of setting yourself a sweeping, unattainable target ('I'm not going to eat any fatty foods ever again!') set one that is manageable and realistic and that you

can measure ('I am not going to eat any crisps for the next month'). If you think you can't possibly avoid crisps for a month, set your goal as a week. Then another. Then another, and so on.

3 **Look for alternatives** If your goal is to stop something – for example, snacking between meals, eating foods that raise levels of bad cholesterol, drinking alcohol or smoking cigarettes – then it helps to give yourself something else to eat/drink/do in its place. The original food or behaviour probably played a specific role for you: it gave you comfort, relaxation, distraction. If, for example, you eat Mars bars when you are bored mid-afternoon, try to schedule a boredom-reducing activity for that time instead: phone a friend, play a game on your computer, watch a DVD, go for a walk. If you try to just stop something, you leave a void. You need to fill that void with something just as pleasurable (only better for you).

4 **Change your environment** It is much harder to 'eat the wrong thing', if the wrong thing isn't waving at you every time you open the fridge or cupboard door. Clear out the food and drink you are trying to avoid (hiding it won't work). Try to remove yourself from temptation: change your walking route so that you no longer go past the bakery, shop online so that you don't see the delicious cheeses at the deli counter, ask a friend to your home instead of meeting in the pub. These changes sound quite drastic, but they need only be short term. Once you have changed your habits and seen the benefits, it will be much easier to resist temptations.

5 **Get support** It is notoriously difficult to make long-term behavioural changes. Your chances of success increase if some-one else can encourage you when you feel like giving up, or help you get back on track when you slip up. If they can make the changes too, even better. It's not always possible, of course,

but if everyone in the home is eating in the same way, your chances of success go up even further.

6 **Reward yourself** Psychological research on learning shows that we learn to repeat the behaviours that have positive consequences. With dietary changes the positive consequences tend to be long term ('My heart will be healthier', 'I will look fabulous at my daughter's wedding next year') rather than immediate. So find other ways to reward yourself in the short term: non-edible treats – buying yourself a bunch of flowers, getting a massage, renting a DVD, or even something small and simple like doing a crossword. As you indulge in your treat, say to yourself, 'This is my reward for ... ' You could even schedule your rewards in your calendar as motivation.

Watch out for Thought Traps

Anyone who has ever tried to control what they eat will know that you're almost bound to slip up sometimes. The danger here is not that bar of chocolate or pint of beer. It's your own pushy, perfectionist thoughts: 'I've failed', 'This is hopeless', 'I always knew I couldn't do it', 'I might as well give up now.' These thoughts are powerful and harsh – and generally unrealistic. They can make the difference between success and failure. The truth is, it's not possible to achieve your aims in life without slips, falls and even great big crashes. It isn't perfection that will get you there, it's resilience – the ability to pick yourself up, dust yourself down and move on. Common eating-related Thought Traps are:

- Catastrophising: 'I've put on two pounds this week, my heart will not be able to cope.'
- Fortune-telling: 'I will never be able to stick to this regime.'
- Filter glasses: 'I ate a slice of chocolate cake today. I am hopeless' (the focus of your attention is on the single incident that went wrong rather than the week of successful healthy eating).

- 'If …, then …' thinking: 'If I don't lose weight every week, then there is no point in continuing with this diet.'

Build your 'case for the defence'

Thought Trap – Filter glasses: 'I ate a slice of chocolate cake today. I am hopeless.'

What is the evidence? You had one slip up, does that make you hopeless? Will one slice set you back hugely? Are you beating yourself up for having one piece of cake when previously you might have eaten several? One slip up does not mean your whole diet is over. You may have actually managed your diet well the rest of the day/week/month. Remind yourself of this.

What are the mitigating circumstances? What was going on when you ate the cake? If someone made it for you, it would have been difficult to refuse. Perhaps you needed comfort or a reward? If you can work out why you ate the cake you may be able to prepare yourself better in future – you may be able to work out how to thank someone for their kindness without eating the cake, or find a different way of rewarding or comforting yourself next time.

Is thinking like this fair or helpful? Focusing on a single mistake and calling yourself hopeless is not going to motivate or encourage you – it's more likely to send you straight back to the cake tin. What's more, ask yourself if you'd ever dream of saying to someone you love, 'Ha, I told you so, I knew you would never manage to keep away from cakes. You have failed at your diet after only a week. You're never going to eat healthily.' Instead, think about what you would say to encourage them ('It's OK, you slipped up, it was really hard, but it was only one tiny mistake. The rest of the week you were incredibly controlled and careful. You can get back on track.'). If you'd say these helpful things to a friend, why not say them to yourself?

TIP

This isn't 'them' imposing things …

… it's *you* taking control.

If you feel put upon or depressed at what you now can't eat, it can help to try to look at the restrictions in a different way. You could view it as a way of you taking back some control over your body. Good nutrition isn't the magic key that will unlock an illness-free future, but it can make a major difference to your health and well-being. Making these changes is a way for you to take charge. You may not always be able to achieve this mindset – and who can blame you – but it can help to try.

❝I made a real effort to eat well – quite simple things really – I cut out takeaways and ready meals and I focused on fresh foods. After a few weeks of this, I began to notice subtle changes – my eyes seemed brighter, I felt more energetic, somehow cleaner inside and I stopped craving sugars and fats. I just felt better, plain and simple. I won't go back to my old habits now. I know this is making a difference and I feel like I've taken control of something.❞

Deena, 58, had a heart attack

TIP

Taking control of giving up smoking

In the same way as taking control of healthy eating, if you are a smoker, whatever health crisis you have just faced, it's obvious that the number-one way to improve your recovery and future health is to *quit*. Giving up smoking is as helpful for people who have already developed smoking-related illnesses as it is for those who haven't yet succumbed to smoking-related disease. Many people do find that their health crisis shocks them into instant 'cold turkey', but if you are still struggling to give up, the first thing to do is get help. Evidence shows that you're more likely to succeed if you follow a structured programme – start with the NHS smoking helpline and the NHS website (see Resources). All the advice on making dietary changes works for quitting smoking too: get personalised advice, set goals, look for alternatives, change your environment, get support, reward yourself, watch out for Thought Traps.

*   *   *   *   *

Eating well really is vital if you want to feel better – stronger, fitter, more energetic – even happier. Making changes to diet or habits can be tough, but these changes will pay off. What goes into your body matters enormously – whatever health issue you have faced. Do give this chapter your best shot. If you instigate your own healthy version of the 'stuffing process' you'll feel the difference. Guaranteed.

NOTES FOR CARERS

'Always have something in readiness; a little beef tea, nicely made and nicely skimmed, a few spoonfuls of jelly ... that may be administered almost as soon as the invalid wishes for it. If obliged to wait a long time, the patient loses the desire to eat, and often turns against the food when brought to him or her.'

Mrs Beeton, *Book of Household Management*, 1861

Preparing food is a tangible way to offer care and support. But it can also be demoralising when your 'nicely made' dish is pushed away, or the 'invalid' won't stick to the doctor's dietary advice. Here are your survival tactics when the going gets tough:

1 **Don't take it personally** Their appetite may be altered for all sorts of reasons, the least of which will be the quality of your cooking.

2 **Learn (or remind yourself) of the principles of healthy eating** This is a key way to boost their health – and your own – and to feel more empowered.

3 **Eat (well) together** Changing eating habits is more likely to be a success if the whole family is in it together. In purely practical terms, if everyone eats the same thing, you won't have to make lots of different dishes.

4 **Expect an adjustment period** If you've lived on takeaways, it can be hard to launch into a plate of curly kale. Expect it to take a while (weeks or even longer) to adjust to dietary changes – and be prepared to persevere. Look for tempting ways to prepare healthy food, rather than forcing down things you find hard to stomach. People can – and do – change their eating habits successfully. But it takes planning and thought and determination.

5 **Don't obsess** Ensuring that your loved one eats the right thing is one of the most obvious ways to gain control over a difficult situation; however, it's easy to feel that you have to control every morsel, or disaster will strike. While it's important to make an effort to follow dietary recommendations, the odd slip up is *not* the end of the world. Expecting perfection is the quickest way to lose faith – and then give up. Instead, make an effort to be 'good enough'.

‘Marlon's heart attack gave our whole family such a shock that we have made big lifestyle changes now. Curries are a monthly treat and I have chucked out our deep-fat fryer. We all try to eat our five-a-day. Marlon is really grateful. He says he has no self-control and it would have been much harder for him if we were still eating the old way.’

Selma, 49, wife of Marlon, 55, who had a heart attack

TEN

STIMULATING AND REVIVING THE CONSTITUTION

EXERCISE AND WELL-BEING

Florence Nightingale wrote that convalescents needed 'absence from head excitement, absence from night hours, proper diet, quiet life, fresh mountain air and different kinds of bathing'. Fresh mountain air and a quiet life might be long shots, but the idea of finding ways to boost your physical and mental well-being is perfectly solid and sensible today. This chapter will show you how.

The wonder drug: exercise

You probably think that those lucky olden-days' convalescents got to lie around for months sipping beef tea and enjoying seaside views without lifting a finger, but this couldn't be further from the truth. The Victorians and Edwardians recognised the value of exercise for recovery. In 1904, Fannie Farmer advised 'a liberal supply of fresh cold air, daily morning cold-water baths, light physical exercise in moderation' for convalescents. Even earlier, in the mid 18th century, doctors recommended sea dips and seaside spas 'for stimulating and reviving the constitution'.

But somewhere along the way, the idea of moving more – rather than less – after ill-health fell out of fashion. Many of us grew up believing that bed rest is best if you have had a health problem. Being told to get moving can be genuinely unsettling.

Bed rest certainly produces results. The only problem is that they're the wrong ones. If you lie around in bed, you achieve muscle weakening, joint stiffening, infections, low mood and bedsores. Today's advice is simple: *get moving* (gradually and safely).

Why exercise?

If exercise were available in pill form, it would be hailed as a miracle cure-all. Among other things, regular exercise can:

- Increase muscle bulk and improve muscle condition.
- Increase strength and endurance.
- Improve coordination and balance.
- Help you lose or maintain weight.
- Lower levels of bad cholesterol.
- Improve mood and outlook.
- Tackle depression.
- Reduce blood pressure.
- Reduce the risk of diabetes.
- Reduce the risk of heart attack or stroke.
- Enhance recovery from cancer, prevent recurrence of cancer, and reduce the risk of developing some cancers.
- Strengthen joints and bones.
- Reduce the risk of osteoporosis.
- Improve immune function.
- Lengthen life.

Despite all these well-documented benefits, we are not all obsessively following the advice from our doctors, physiotherapists or the Department of Health when it comes to exercise. One problem is that these health benefits aren't very obvious. You don't wake up thinking, 'Wow, my cholesterol's looking good today.' It is therefore easy to get demoralised, distracted or just plain bored when trying to exercise – particularly if it is hard, painful and tiring.

It can therefore help to focus on the benefits of exercise that *are* more immediate and noticeable. With regular exercise you can:

- Have more control over your body – you will be able to get around better and feel more confident.
- Feel less tired and get more done.
- Be less anxious or stressed.
- Feel happier (exercise improves mood; it is as effective in treating mild-to-moderate depression as antidepressant drugs are).
- Feel better about how your body looks – and therefore, feel better about yourself in general.
- Sleep better (as long as you don't exercise just before bed).
- Have more brain power.
- Feel and look great!

EXERCISE VERSUS ACTIVITY

Exercise is something more organised that you plan, and then do, very regularly – an exercise class, sports, gym visits, walking, swimming. You have goals, and you gradually increase what you can do. Activity, on the other hand, is simply anything physical that involves movement. Activity is definitely something to build into your life. But it is easy to kid yourself that you are being active when in fact you are quite sedentary, so beware of thinking, 'I went to the shop – that counts.' To get health benefits, you must increase your heart rate and reach a point where you are warm and mildly out of breath (see opposite for how much and how often). If you know you'll never stick at gyms, classes or structure, it's fine to just think in terms of building up your daily activity. But be brutally honest with yourself: make sure that you set goals and increase whatever you do.

How much?

Always talk to your doctor before you start an exercise regime. It is important to establish what is appropriate for you to do given your age, and physical abilities. Make sure you also ask your medical team about any warning signs that you should not ignore while exercising. Write down the answers to these questions. If you have a clear list of 'symptoms' to watch out for, you will be far less likely to panic at the first twinge – and quit.

In order to stay physically healthy, you should aim to be active for some time every day.

The current government recommendations

- At least 2½ hours of 'moderate intensity' physical activity over the course of one week. Moderate intensity means something that raises your heart and breathing rate, makes you break into a light sweat and get warmer, or slightly red (you should still be able to carry on a conversation while you're doing it). Activities such as brisk walking, cycling on flat ground, water aerobics, pushing a lawnmower, rollerblading and dancing fit into the 'moderate activity' category.

- Or 75 minutes (1¼ hours) of vigorous activity, such as running or a game of singles tennis every week.

- Your activity should be done in minimum bouts of 10 minutes at a time (but ideally should build up to 30-minute sessions five days a week).

- As well as your activity, you should do something that strengthens your muscles at least twice a week. This should involve weight-bearing and resistance. Lifting weights in the gym, push-ups, sit-ups, intensive gardening, such as digging, carrying heavy shopping, or some forms of yoga and Pilates all count.

- Older adults who are at risk of falls are also encouraged to carry out balance and coordination activities twice a week: t'ai chi, yoga and Pilates are all good at strengthening, balance and coordination.

Getting to this level takes time – if you try to do too much too fast you could cause yourself an injury or, at the very least, put yourself off trying. Always make sure that you build up very gradually – to whatever goal you have set for yourself. These guidelines are the government's goals for healthy people but, of course, they may be completely unrealistic for you. The main thing is to think about building some form of activity into your life – even if it has to be done from your armchair! (For more information, see Resources.)

TIP

Rename it ...

If the word 'exercise' catapults you back to standing miserably on the school sports pitch, then change the name – call it activity, getting into the garden, 'my walk round the block', tennis, Friday-night dancing – but whatever it is that you call it, try to build it into your life.

Why it's hard to do all this when you've been unwell

Exercise can be hard to do even when you are perfectly healthy. Only 40 per cent of men and 28 per cent of women in the UK currently hit the government targets (and in the 65 to 74 age bracket, this figure plummets to 17 per cent of men and 13 per cent of women). If you've faced a health crisis, this sort of goal can seem nonsensical. It may be that even the smallest movement is a major challenge to you right now. And even if you are mobile, you are probably coping with reduced fitness levels, muscle loss or weakness, and lowered energy levels. You are also likely to be grappling with a lack of information and perhaps with pain and fear too. All of this can make regular exercise seem impossible.

> ❝I felt completely daunted by the idea of exercising after my heart surgery. It was so much harder than recovering from gall bladder surgery ten years before. I was aware of my age, of my general lower level of fitness, I had arthritis in my knees which made moving painful and, above all, I was scared that exercise might damage my heart or dislodge the new valve.❞
> **Laurence, 65, had heart valve replacement surgery**

This is completely fair enough; however, the answer is not to just give up. You have to tackle both your mind and your body so that this becomes achievable – and enjoyable.

Tackling the fear factor

Fear is a huge barrier to exercise after a health crisis. Common fears include:

- Fear of making things worse physically; for example, triggering another heart attack or stroke, causing further injury or pain.

- Fear of failure: not getting back to a previous level of fitness, not meeting your own goals.

- Fear of being seen by others (and looking silly).

- Fear of facing your limitations.

- Fear of the unknown (even if you were once a sports fanatic, exercising after a serious health problem can be an unknown).

Given the complexity of these emotions, it's hardly surprising if a few brief words of medical advice, or a slim information leaflet, don't make you want to leap up and join the British Athletics Squad.

Ways to tackle these fears

Get expert and specific advice Your age, your interests, your previous levels of fitness and activity, your medical history, your current physical status, are just a few of the variables that count when finding the right form of exercise. Start with your medical team, or ask for a referral to a physiotherapist. Your local council should also have a list of many of the groups and services available for people who want to start exercising after a health problem.

Get support You are more likely to stick at it if you have company and support. At hospital or community rehabilitation courses you'll meet others in similar situations, and this can be invaluable. Don't be put off by the 'group' thing – you don't have to bare your soul or discuss your childhood, you'll just be guided through a specialised exercise programme.

Some health charities have local groups where you can meet others in similar situations. Or you could find a local exercise group or class. Local gyms or leisure centres may offer personal fitness trainers – some will have additional training in supporting people recovering from illness and injury (some local authorities and councils have special schemes or subsidised gym membership for people recovering from illness who want to rebuild their fitness).

❝I go to an Age UK class. It is one of the highlights of my week. The lady who runs the class is always coming up with new things for us to do. I feel safe with her supervising us, she can tell us if we are doing the exercises right or not.❞

Greta, 78, had a hip replacement

Find an 'exercise buddy' Your partner, a friend or colleague, who will join in your exercise plan, can make a huge difference to whether you stick at something.

Make a plan and set goals You might start out full of good intentions, but any slight change or problem can bring your plan crashing down. Before you start, sit down with a pen and paper, and set yourself SMART (Specific, Measurable, Achievable, Realistic and Time-limited) goals. (See page 115 for how to do this.)

TIP

Overprotective supporters

While it's great to have someone rooting for you, encouraging you and bolstering your efforts to be more active, It's important to recognise that some supporters – particularly loved ones – can be overprotective. They say things like, 'But you look so tired, why not give it a miss tonight?' or 'You should just take it easy, don't push yourself like this.' Share your activity plan, reassure them that you've had medical advice and you know what signs to watch out for. Don't let an overprotective 'supporter' hold you back.

Warm up and cool down

A warm up and cool down will help to prevent injury and stiffness. Try this five-minute warm up/cool down at the start and end of your exercise session – gently, if you are not very flexible:

1 Move your head from shoulder to shoulder.

2 Pull your chin to your chest and then tip your head back again.

3 Shrug your shoulders.

4 Hold your hands together in front of you and lift your arms above your head. Now hold your hands together behind your back and raise them as high as you can.

5 Circle your feet (one at a time and sitting on a chair if balance is tricky).

6 Pull your toes up towards your shin so that you stretch the calf muscle in the back of your leg (again sitting down if balance is difficult).

7 Stand with your feet wide and let your hands slide down your legs towards the floor so that you stretch your hamstring muscles at the back of your thighs.

TIP

Try walking

If you can manage it, walking is a great way to become more active. It offers cardiovascular fitness benefits and weight-bearing benefits (stronger muscles and bones). It is also very adaptable – you can start walking slowly, for short periods, and build up so that you go faster for longer. You can do it anywhere. You don't need special equipment. It is free. It gets you outside. You can build it into your day, using it to get from A to B, rather than feeling like you are forcing yourself to go to a gym. Try to build up to walking for at least 30 minutes a day, although breaking this up into smaller bursts even of 10 minutes at a time, is fine.

If you are worried or uncertain of your abilities, you could start, for example, by walking 5 minutes out to a fixed point, and then 5 minutes back home, for the first week. Then increase this by 5 minutes each week. Do it by time, rather than distance, so that you aren't stuck somewhere, exhausted and unable to get home. If you know you can definitely walk for 10 minutes, you can set off confident that you'll get home again.

Chairobics – or what to do if you can't walk

If exercise is the 'wonder drug' and walking is the most valuable exercise you can do when recovering from illness or injury, then what happens if you can't walk? Is this wonder drug for other people not you? The answer, luckily, is no!

If you can't walk at the moment, you certainly should have had advice from a doctor or physiotherapist about how best to avoid muscle wasting and maintain good blood circulation. If you can't remember what your doctor said, don't just give up. See if you still have the leaflets. If not, you could get in touch with the physiotherapy department again – you might be able to arrange a home visit or at least have the information sent to you again.

Many exercises can be done from bed or in a chair. A physiotherapist will be able to advise you on how to do this, but so called 'chairobics' can include: rolling your shoulders up, back and down; arm raises; fist clenching then releasing; finger stretching; bicep curls; leg lifting; foot pointing; buttock squeezing or knee bending. Adding light weights (a piece of fruit, a bottle of water, a can of beans) or Therabands (resistance ribbons) can help build up your strength.

All the ideas about how to start and maintain activity apply whether you're rollerblading or doing 'chairobics' (or even 'bedercise'). Get information and support; plan and set SMART goals; challenge your Thought Traps and reward yourself. You can still benefit from exercise even if you aren't romping around outdoors, so don't give up, don't skip this chapter and think, 'This is not about me.' Yes – this is about you too!

⁶When I first got home I was bedridden, but the exercises I did from bed helped build up my muscle strength and I progressed out of bed and into a wheelchair. It was slow and frustrating at times, but I set myself little goals and that kept me motivated. I had to learn from my physiotherapist how to stand up, but I can now walk around my kitchen and living room. I gave myself a reward when I stopped being bed-bound – I went in my wheelchair to a football match. I've always supported my team, and getting back there in person was overwhelming. It was a wonderful day, another tick in the box.⁹

Bernie, 72, had a stroke

How to build up what you do

At the Battle Creek Sanitarium, Michigan, in the late 19th century, John Harvey Kellogg had people out in the cold air doing postural exercises, calisthenics, gymnastics and swimming. There were hydrotherapies, massage, dietary changes – and rest – all in the name of health and well-being.

Exercise, of course, does not have to be exhausting and painful, but effort is important. It can be hard to know how to build up your activity levels safely and effectively. But one good trick is to think in terms of how much 'effort' you are putting into your exercise. Rehabilitation experts have developed a 'perceived effort scale' for this:

PERCEIVED EFFORT SCALE	
Exercise effort	**The way you feel**
0 Nothing	Able to sing/whistle. Activity easily performed
1 Very little	
2	
3 Moderate	Slow to comfortable walk. You can talk easily. You feel warmer with some muscle effort. Breathing will be slightly faster and deeper
4	
5 Comfortably strong	Brisk to fast walk. You will feel warmer and feel muscle effort
6	Stronger vigorous exercise. Difficulty talking. Breathing hard
7 Strong	Short of breath
8	
9 Very strong indeed	All-out effort, which is unable to be maintained
10	Exhausted. STOP!

How to use this scale

At first, as you begin to increase your activity levels (using SMART goals), keep within 3–5 on your effort scale: you're comfortable and can speak easily as you exercise.

Then, when you feel that this is almost too easy – and this can be days or weeks into your exercise programme – see if you can start to increase your effort levels so that you are working between levels 5–7 as you exercise (you are getting even warmer, breathing faster and can feel your muscles working hard).

This will gradually push your body, in a safe and controlled way, so that your fitness and strength increase.

> ## TIP
>
> ### Stick at it
>
> It can take up to four weeks for you to see any changes whatsoever to your fitness or energy levels, so stick at it. It is also worth recognising that the first few times are likely to feel really hard – you may feel sore and achy afterwards. But persevere – you will feel less sore and achy as your body adapts.
>
> ### What to do if it feels 'wrong'
>
> As we pointed out on earlier in this chapter, you should always consult your doctor or medical team before you start any new form of exercise or activity to make sure that it's appropriate and safe. If something you are doing just feels 'wrong' then stop, and get medical advice before you continue. But don't give up on the idea of exercise. To get those wonder-drug payoffs you will need to – gradually and safely – increase your effort levels. This may be worrying at first. But it is fine to take it slow and to get expert advice or reassurance along the way. You may well be monitoring your bodily sensations more closely – any twinge, ache or pain, change in temperature or breathing rate might seem very noticeable. Don't panic. Bear in mind your list of 'warning signs' (see page 241). But equally don't ignore your alarm bells. If you are uncertain, check with your doctor.

Tackling your thoughts

Some Thought Traps will stop you from trying exercise, others will get in your way when you have begun. Tackling your Thought Traps therefore needs to become as much a part of your routine as slipping on your walking shoes or meeting your 'exercise buddy' at the scheduled time. Common exercise-related Thought Traps include:

- All-or-nothing thinking: 'I'm never going to stick to this, so there's no point trying', 'I'm not an exercise person.'

- Labelling: 'I'm far too disabled/weak/pathetic/fat to walk that far/start swimming/join an exercise class.'

- Catastrophising: 'If I exercise, I'll do myself terrible damage', 'I'm going to rip my wound apart', 'I'll have another heart attack if I walk fast.'

Build your 'case for the defence'

Example: Thought Trap – All or nothing: 'I'm not an exercise person.'

What's the evidence? You may not have been an exercise person before, but there were probably times when you were active. Did you walk to pick up your paper, do heavy gardening or housework, climb the stairs at work? What exercise have you managed before? Even if you were not 'sporty', did you enjoy walking, swimming or cycling? Were you 'too busy' to fit formal exercise into your life before, but is the situation different now? Were you held back from exercise before by lack of knowledge or fear? Might you be able to overcome these, if you can find the right support for yourself?

What are the mitigating circumstances? You may have been more 'active' than you give yourself credit for. Just because you didn't like team or organised sports doesn't mean you were a total 'couch potato'. Even if you were, you may now have more motivation to change your lifestyle. Your life has changed, you've had a health crisis, no one is expecting you to leap from your sick bed onto an athletics track. You need to take this active approach gently, build up gradually and get support.

Is thinking like this fair or helpful? It is not fair or helpful to write yourself off as 'not an exercise person'. This kind of thinking is more likely to stop you from trying. Think about other changes you may have made to your life in the past. Tell yourself you can do this too. If you're expecting yourself to win an Olympic gold rather than just get going, this isn't fair either. Nor is comparing yourself to people who haven't been through what you've been through. It is more helpful to say encouraging things to yourself – the sort of things you'd say to someone you love ('I'm going to give this my best shot', 'I'm doing well', 'I've made a start', 'This is a great first step').

'Taking the Air' – why getting outside is good

The Canadian Medical Association announced in 1932 that convalescent homes should 'provide ample sitting rooms and solaria. Sun porches on each floor and perhaps the roof ... Grounds should be ample. Woodland walks, a small golf course, archery, bowling, tennis and other outdoor facilities should be developed.' They were right. Researchers at Essex University have shown that exercise is even more beneficial to mood if it is done outside in a natural environment. Scandinavian researchers, meanwhile, have established that hospital patients who have an open, interesting view from their window recover faster than those who look at a brick wall.

Even if your chosen exercise is indoors (swimming, for example, or the gym) try to plan daily outings – anywhere that you can see greenery will do. If you cannot physically get outside then you can find ways of bringing nature inside – even small, slightly silly ones. Looking at books or magazines or websites with images of the outdoors, having flowers or plants by your chair or bed, or even just sitting by a window where you can glimpse a tree or two.

&Once I was mobile enough to get out of the flat I took my walking frame and went to my local park which, luckily, is just next to me. It felt like a release from prison. I could walk slowly and then sit on a bench. I saw the trees and flowers; I knew it was spring. It was hard to go back home! 9

Mary, 48, broke her leg in a car crash

Reward yourself

Exercise in itself becomes rewarding – it floods you with endorphins (the body's 'feel-good' chemicals) and gives you a sense of achievement. But sometimes the benefits of exercise itself aren't immediate enough. It helps to find ways to reward yourself – finish your walk by going to a friend's home; put some money into your treat/holiday pot each time you go swimming; treat yourself to your favourite TV programme after the gym, or buy a magazine on the way home. Crucially, make sure to tell yourself that you are getting this treat because you deserve it after your exercise.

KEEP ON GOING

If you have been doing a formal rehabilitation programme and it is coming to a close, try to think carefully about how you'll stay active now. If you just think, 'Oh, I'll stay active somehow', you might not. You have to make it happen by finding the right activity, setting goals, getting support and rewarding yourself.

&In the ten years since my heart attack I have continued to take a daily walk, go to the hospital gym every week and the heart

---

support group once a month. It helps me to feel that I am keeping
up to date with all the latest developments in coronary care and
also that I am exercising in the best way possible. 🤟

Derek, 77, had a heart attack

Ways to boost your well-being

Boosting your 'well-being' probably sounds a bit woolly. Well-
being goes beyond being physically stronger and fitter. It is
about feeling contented and effective (whatever your circumstances). People with high levels of well-being are also
resilient – they hold up well when faced with challenges.

You might be thinking, 'Yeah, lucky them', but what is interesting about well-being is that it can be learnt.

Studies show that well-being isn't dependent on past experience or genes (although these can certainly either help or
hinder). It is based on patterns of behaviour and styles of thinking. Scientists have identified five factors – dubbed 'GREAT
behaviours' that promote well-being:

1 Giving

2 Relating/connecting

3 Exercise

4 Awareness

5 Trying things out/learning

To boost your well-being – and therefore feel an awful lot
better whatever you are dealing with – you want to aim to
include all five of these GREAT behaviours in your day. Think
of them as your well-being 'five-a-day'.

1 Giving

One of the quickest ways to feel better is to be kind, helpful and generous. This is not pious lecturing – it is backed by good scientific data. Recent neuro-imaging research has shown that cooperating with and giving to others stimulates the 'reward centre' in the brain. Result: you feel better. You may feel as if your life right now is more about taking than giving – and there's nothing much you can do about this; however, the well-being studies show that it's not just the big things like running a scout troupe that can make you feel great. Small acts of 'giving' work too – saying thank you, smiling at a friend, making a cup of tea for someone, holding a door open for someone, letting someone on the bus ahead of you, listening to or offering help to a friend in any small way.

> ❝I go to check on my neighbour every day. She's a lady in her nineties and all alone. I like to visit her just before it gets dark. We chat and I make sure she has a warm drink. It works well for both of us. I notice on the odd day that I can't get to her I worry about her and I feel like I haven't done my good deed of the day.❞
>
> **Margaret, 63, had heart bypass surgery**

2 Relating to or connecting with others

People who score higher on psychologists' well-being tests have stronger, happier relationships with family, friends, colleagues and community. Although you may not be able to solve all your 'issues', one good trick is to simply try to 'be there' more. When you are with someone, focus on them. Put away your laptop, turn your phone to silent, listen to the answer when you ask a question. You could try having lunch with a colleague rather than at your desk, tracking down an old friend, or simply saying hello to people in your neighbourhood.

Spending time at your place of worship or a club of interest to you can help you to connect to others. You may be thinking, 'I don't have time to join clubs or hang out chatting to strangers!' Fair enough: you may not have time or inclination to run a British Heart Foundation Shop or organise a prayer meeting, but the time commitment involved in simply focusing on the person you're with is pretty minimal. And it will pay dividends.

❝I joined a knitting group – it sounds bonkers for a man in his forties – but it's been utterly fantastic. Before, I was working hard, then going out drinking. It was doing me no good and I was worn out. Now, I meet great people who I'd never have known – some older, some my age – I have learned something genuinely satisfying and creative, and quite useful, and I find it completely relaxing. I look forward to my group every week – I'd say it's my lifeline!❞

Stan, 47, had a burst appendix

3 Exercise

This is a vital one of your five-a-day – another great reason to take exercise seriously.

❝I walk on the Fells or in the Lake District as often as I can, at least twice a week. Having a view takes me out of myself. I take that view home with me in my mind and it lasts till I get back there the next time.❞

David, 55, had a cerebral aneurism

4 Awareness

It is easy to spend your life looking back or ahead and completely bypassing the here and now. Concentrating on the present moment can make you feel calmer, more grounded and accepting. Reliable scientific studies show that this is a highly effective way to increase your well-being. Mindfulness is a great approach to living in the present. A mindfulness course is ideal, but books, CDs and apps can also help you to develop your 'here and now' skills (see Resources).

Try this: two simple mindfulness exercises

Mindful eating Think about your main meal of the day. How often have you wolfed it down, perhaps adding a glass of wine or pint of beer, finishing without really having paid any attention? At your next meal, slow down: pay attention to the taste, aromas, textures, temperatures. Notice how your body feels and responds. This will make you enjoy your meal far more, and may stop your mind from racing.

Or:

Mindful walk Instead of going from A to B, try to notice what you can see, hear, feel, smell. How does your body feel? Notice the swishing of the air, temperature changes, your footfall, the movement of your joints. Familiar scenes may seem boring, but look at the detail – examine paving stones, plants, a spider's web. This can anchor you in the present moment, and help you to appreciate and accept the way things are. You can do this with other daily activities too – showering, brushing your teeth, even just sitting on the sofa. Examining your senses as well as your thoughts, emotions and physical sensations can help you to 'wake up to the world around you'.

TIP

Count your blessings

It does sound Pollyanna-ish, and it's infuriating to be told by someone how lucky you are. It doesn't always help to think about people who are worse off than you, either. But if you can take time to think about things that are good in your life – even during the dark days – you will feel less fraught. Thinking about good moments – however brief they are – also helps you become more aware of them as they happen.

Try this: catch a happy thought

- At the end of each day write down at least one moment that was pleasurable for you (more if you want to).

- Note down what was happening, what you thought and felt and how writing it down makes you feel and think now.

- Noticing this level of detail will make you more aware next time there is a positive moment – it will also simply help you to end your day feeling happier.

5 Try new things

Studies show that lifelong learning is really good for your well-being. This doesn't mean signing up for self-improving evening classes (though they can be fantastic sources of well-being). It is simply about trying new things. Sheila Pim noted in her *Convalescent's Handbook* that 'If you make rugs or nets, or even learn such a frivolous craft as paper folding, it keeps at bay that dreary feeling of a completely wasted day.' You might want to try something beyond paper folding – signing up for a creative writing course, learning a new language or playing an instrument, for example. But small things are great too – cooking a new recipe, reading a new book, discovering a new function on your phone. Or, you could test yourself socially – do a presentation at work, invite a new friend round for lunch.

Some of the more basic skills might also be 'new' in a sense now too – walking after a knee replacement, bathing after a stroke, going back to work after surgery are all, in a sense, new skills. Try to recognise these achievements. Reward yourself for them.

> ❝The only thing my consultant said to me at the end of my treatment was that I should visit places I had never been to and take up new interests and hobbies so that I would never make comparisons to the pre-cancerous me. I have moved to the coast and taken up painting and I have a deep sense of contentment I never ever expected at this stage of my life.❞
>
> **Faith, 61, had thyroid cancer**

You've got to laugh

Humour really can be 'the best medicine'. Many people find that as a coping strategy, nothing beats it. Elaine, wife of Malcolm, 67, who had a cardiac defibrillator fitted, describes the cardiac rehabilitation course he goes to as 'his dicky-ticker club'. She teases him that he needs to put the life insurance papers at the front of his filing cabinet. Hywel, 31, who had testicular cancer, goes to a comedy club night with friends at least once a month.

> ❝When I am in that club laughing my head off, nothing bothers me. I relax completely and let go. For a short

> while I can forget what I have been through – it's my
> main coping strategy and if I'm at home I will always try
> to find a comedy show to watch on TV.

Studies into the actual physical effects of humour and laughter on health are a bit controversial (some studies seem to show that laughter reduces pain and enhances the immune system, but the methods of these studies have been criticised); however, there is no doubt that if you can laugh about it, you'll probably feel better – at least for a bit. Humour can also be incredibly bonding. Some couples find they can't talk about their fears, but they can laugh together, and that works just as well.

> Before I went in to have my kidney removed I made
> my husband write over the healthy one, in black marker
> pen, "Not this one!" It cracked us up – we were literally
> crying with laughter. The consultant didn't find it funny,
> but it got us through what could have been a very grim
> morning.
>
> **Sue, 40, had a kidney removed**

* * * * *

This chapter has taken you through well-being strategies that will make you feel an awful lot better, from the inside out, whatever you are coping with. Developing new habits is rarely simple or easy, not least when you are battling health issues. But doing so will pay off, massively. The strategies in this chapter are not the suggestions of a couple of airy-fairy do-gooders: every single one is rooted in solid scientific research. This means they actually work. And they will work for you, too, if you give them a go.

NOTES FOR CARERS

'There is more excitement about Bath-chairing – especially if you are not used to the exhilarating exercise – than might appear to the casual observer. A sense of danger ... is ever present to the mind of the occupant ... Every vehicle that passes he expects is going to run into him; and he never finds himself ascending or descending a hill without immediately beginning to speculate upon his chances, supposing ... that the weak-kneed controller of his destiny should let go.'

Jerome K Jerome, 'On Being Idle',
*Idle Thoughts of an Idle Fellow***, 1889**

The value of exercising after illness or injury – whether in a bath chair or on both legs – is one of the most important messages in this book; however, as a carer, your position can be very tricky indeed. There is a fine line between encouragement and nagging. You may find yourself worrying about health and safety issues. And it can be deeply frustrating if your loved one either won't do their exercise or seems to be jeopardising their health by doing too much, or the wrong thing. It can also be very difficult to encourage someone to enhance their own 'well-being'. At times you will feel that you are in control of the 'bath chair' – easing your loved one at a steady pace in the right direction. At others you may feel distinctly weak-kneed about your role, patience or efficacy. You may even (though you would never do it) want to push that bath chair off a cliff.

Here are some things that will make all this less fraught:

1 **Inform yourself** For your own peace of mind, it is important that you really do understand how exercise should work in this situation. Try to talk to your loved one's medical team about this, and read any exercise leaflets or materials they have. If there is an appropriate health charity, read the exercise section on their website (or call their helpline). If

possible, you want to get specific advice: how much exercise is good, what sort of exercise is appropriate. Also, establish very clearly what warning signs you should look out for – this way you won't panic every time they say they're tired, or achy (see page 241).

2 **Agree on your role** How much are you going to 'remind' them to exercise or rest? In what way? See if you can come up with an agreement on what will work to prompt and encourage the person you are caring for, without causing tension and frustration for both of you.

3 **Find an 'exercise buddy' for your loved one** It doesn't have to be you. Exercise will do you good too, of course, but if you are already overloaded or you simply need a break from each other, this is something you could consider 'delegating' to a willing friend or relative.

4 **Find ways to be active and social together** Of course, what you choose to do will depend on your shared interests and any physical restrictions, but do think outside the box – a walking group, a dance class, and so on.

5 **Appreciate the small things every day** This simple strategy can be enormously helpful as you go through the daily 'grind' of caring for someone. Try to be aware of the world around you: study the colour of the sky, the silhouettes on the horizon; recognise how great it feels getting into a hot bath or listening to birdsong. Contemplate this sort of thing for yourself, but also talk about these 'small pleasures' with the person you are caring for. It is surprising how the little things add up to a sense of greater happiness and contentment, whatever else is going on. Don't force it, but if you feel it, then share it.

6 **Try not to be overprotective** You may well want to wrap the person up in cotton wool after what you have all been

through, but remember that many of their GREAT behaviours (see page 254) will involve them getting out there and doing things for themselves and for other people. You may think they're better off tucked safely in the (metaphorical) bath chair with you gripping the handles and steering, but sometimes you have to let them get up and go.

❝We got Mum a little dog to cheer her up after her illness. We got him as company for her, but of course he has really helped her with exercise. She has to take him out twice a day. At the start my wife or I went with her, but she is much steadier and more confident now, so we only accompany her when we all go for a family walk. Another unexpected advantage is that she has made lots of "dog" friends in the park ❞

Chris, 43, son of Rose, 72, who had pneumonia

CONCLUSION

❛I knew that I felt better when, seven years after my collapse, I booked a summer holiday abroad without checking how close the hotel was to a hospital.❜

Melanie, 66, had a heart attack

We've come a long way since the days of bath chairs and heroin-laced 'tonics'. But what is surprising is that, despite miraculous medical advances, many of the emotional challenges of ill health are essentially unchanged. We still need to get back our confidence and *joie de vivre* after a serious illness or injury. Whether the treatment involved hi-tech lasers or leeches, we still need to adapt to changes; communicate our needs and fears; rebuild our confidence and strength – and move on with our lives.

Many people never get back to exactly where they were before. They have physical, practical or emotional challenges to cope with. But they find ways to manage these challenges, and to live a fulfilling life – on their own terms. Nobody is suggesting that this is easy. It may take a long time. It can certainly take effort, but it has happened to other people – and it can happen to you too, whatever you are dealing with.

We hope this book has helped you to recognise that feeling better isn't just a physical challenge: there are emotional 'tasks' too. If you are finding this process slow, painful and difficult, you are far from unusual. But try to remind yourself that 'feeling better' is not set in stone. Only you can know what 'feeling better' really means.

This, then, is your 'How to Feel Better' kit – you can carry it with you (on your Kindle, in your bag or in your head), picking out the coping skills you need, as and when you need them. You can do this now, but you can also come back to it again in the future – because your needs and concerns are bound to change.

If you are a carer, we hope this book has shown you that your feelings matter too. Your caring role, while undeniably challenging, can be manageable, if you have some strategies to hand.

The snippets about convalescence in the past aren't just here to amuse you (although anything that makes you smile can't be bad). They are here to show you how much of the wisdom and common sense in that supposedly outdated idea of 'convalescence' is now borne out by scientific evidence. It can't hurt to keep those wise Edwardians or Victorians in mind as you focus on feeling better. They took this seriously – and so should we.

George Bernard Shaw once wrote: 'I enjoy convalescence. It is the part that makes the illness worthwhile.' Although you might not go that far, we hope that our 'modern art of convalescence' has at least helped you to understand that feeling better isn't something that just happens out of the blue. It's something you can influence. You can make this happen – so, over to you . . .

RESOURCES

UK
Help with common health conditions – for sufferers and carers

NHS Choices
Website: www.nhs.uk
The UK's biggest health website providing information to help people understand their condition and make choices about their health.

British Heart Foundation
Website: www.bhf.org.uk
Heart Helpline: 0300 330 3311
The UK's leading heart charity, offering a wealth of information and support for anything heart-related.

Stroke Association
Website: www.stroke.org.uk
Helpline: 0303 303 3100
Information and support on any issue to do with stroke – for people who have had a stroke, as well as their families, friends and carers. There are local groups and an online community.

Health talk online
Website: www.healthtalkonline.org
Videos and interview transcripts of more than 2000 people, sharing their experiences of living with over 60 health-related conditions and illnesses. Provides support and information, helping patients and families to benefit from the experiences of others.

Macmillan Cancer Support
Website: www.macmillan.org.uk
Tel: 0808 808 0000
Provides information, a telephone helpline, post-treatment courses and local support. Also offers information and support to family and friends.

Maggie's Cancer Caring Centres
Website: www.maggiescentres.org.uk
Tel: 0300 123 1801
Provides a website, information, online support and local drop-in centres
close to many UK cancer centres. Offers post-treatment, relaxation and
stress-management courses.

Carers UK
Website: www.carersuk.org
Tel: 0808 808 7777
Support and advice for carers on all aspects of caring including great
information resources and ways to find local support.

Worries, Anxiety and Depression

Money Worries
National Debtline: 0808 808 4000
This helpline provides free, confidential and independent advice on how to
deal with debt problems

International Stress Management Association
Website: www.isma.org.uk
Tel: 0845 680 7083
Information about all types of stress, with stress-relief tips and a referral
service for stress counsellors.

Mindfulness
Website: www.bemindful.co.uk
Introduction to mindfulness, including ways to find a course near you.

Depression Alliance
Website: www.depressionalliance.org
Tel: 0845 123 2320
Wide range of information and support for anyone suffering from
depression, or their loved ones.

Living Life to the Full
Website: www.lttf.com
A free online 'life skills' programme based on cognitive-behavioural
principles. The course covers how to tackle the stresses and challenges we
face in everyday life, including anxiety and depression.

Mind
Website: www.mind.org.uk
Tel: 0300 123 3393
Information and support for people with mental health problems and their
families.

The Royal College of Psychiatrists
Website: www.rcpsych.ac.uk/expertadvice/problems
Provides a range of leaflets and online advice on a large number of
emotional issues, as well as lists of organisations and contacts that can help.

Helpguide
Website: www.helpguide.org
Information about mental health difficulties and simple, expert,
practical advice on how to cope. Covers healthy lifestyle and ageing
topics as well.

Samaritans
Website: www.samaritans.org
Tel: 0845 790 9090
Phone and face-to-face support for anyone who feels suicidal or despairing.
Branches all over the UK open 24 hours a day, every day of the year.

Nutrition and General Health

The British Nutrition Foundation
Website: www.nutrition.org.uk
The website has a 'healthy living' section which includes the basics of good
nutrition.

NHS
Website: www.nhs.uk/livewell/healthy-eating
The NHS website has good basic information about eating a balanced diet.

NHS Smoking Helpline
Tel: 0800 022 4332
NHS stop smoking resource that has helped thousands to quit.

Patient UK
Website: www.patient.co.uk
Organisation offering information for patients on a range of health
services. The website has sections on various conditions, with details of
support groups, information leaflets, and links to related organisations.

The National Sleep Foundation
Website: www.sleepfoundation.org
This American website is a good resource, offering sleep facts, information
on sleep problems and good sleep tips.

The Mayo Clinic
Website: www.mayoclinic.com
A hospital website with a detailed fitness and healthy living section.

Active Places

Website: www.activeplaces.com
Allows you to find sports facilities in your local area, or use the name and address of a specific facility to find out more information.

Walking for Health

Email: ramblers@ramblers.org.uk
Tel: 0300 060 2287
Set up by Macmillan Cancer Care and The Ramblers, this is a programme of local walking groups – open to anyone at all (not just those with or after cancer!). Suitable for walkers at all levels.

Relationships and Sex

Relate

Website: www.relate.org.uk
Tel: 0300 100 1234
National organisation offering information and expert counselling on relationships and sex – by phone, online, or in person.

The Institute of Psychosexual Medicine

Website: www.itm.org.uk
Help in finding a doctor who specialises in sexual problems (both physical and emotional).

Online Sex and Relationships Therapy

Website: www.sextherapyonline.org
Online help from trained therapists, allows you to remain anonymous and can be fitted around a busy schedule.

Well-being

Do It

Website: www.do-it.org.uk
A national online resource offering volunteering opportunities – helps you to find opportunities in your area and apply for them online.

IVO

Website: www.ivo.org
An online social network that connects community-minded people who want to volunteer, and provides information on opportunities all over the UK.

Volunteering England

Website: www.volunteering.org.uk
Can put you in touch with your local volunteering centre.

South Africa

The Heart and Stroke Foundation South Africa
Website: www.heartfoundation.co.za
As well as information on heart disease and stroke, has good guidelines on food, lifestyle, exercise and general health.

Stroke Survivors Foundation
Website: www.strokesurvivors.org.za
Speak-to-a-stroke-survivor line: 082 889 1800
A national network providing post-discharge rehabilitation and support for stroke survivors, their families and caregivers.

The South African Depression and Anxiety Group
Website: www.sadag.org
Comprehensive mental health information and resources to help sufferers and their families.

The Cancer Association of South Africa
Website: www.cansa.org.za
Tel: 0800 22 66 22
Provides information and support for people with cancer.

South African Federation for Mental Health
Website: www.safmh.org.za
Suicide Crisis Line 8am–8pm: 0800 567 567
South Africa's largest mental health support and advocacy group offering information on mental health conditions such as depression, sleep problems and anxiety.

Australia

Heart Foundation
Website: www.heartfoundation.org.au
Tel: 1300 362 787
Information and support on cardiovascular health, including guidelines for healthy living and activity.

The Stroke Foundation
Website: www.strokefoundation.com.au
Strokeline: 1800 787 653
Information, advice and support for anyone who has had a stroke, and their families or carers.

Relationships Australia
Website: www.relationships.org.au
Support and counselling for relationship problems. This has an interactive map that allows you to find local support.

Cancer Australia
Website: www.canceraustralia.gov.au
Australian government website with information on all aspects of cancer,
including local cancer support organisations.

The Samaritans
Website: www.thesamaritans.org.au
24/7 crisis line: 08 9381 5555
Non-judgemental emotional support for the despairing and suicidal.

Australian Government's healthy eating advice
Website: www.eatforhealth.gov.au

New Zealand
Heart Foundation
Website: www.heartfoundation.org.nz
Information and advice on all aspects of heart disease.

Stroke Foundation of New Zealand
Website: www.stroke.org.nz
Info Line: 0800 STROKE (78 76 53)
Information and support for sufferers and their families.

Relationships Aotearoa
Website: www.relationshipsaotearoa.org.nz
Couples, workplace, family and personal counselling and advice.

Mental Health Foundation of New Zealand
Website: www.mentalhealth.org.nz
Information and support on mental health issues including depression.
Lists local numbers to phone in a crisis.

Samaritans
Website: www.samaritans.org.nz
Tel: 0800 726 666 (this number is available for callers from the Lower
North Island, Christchurch and the West Coast only. Callers from other
regions please phone 0800 211 211 or 04 472 3676)

Cancer Society of New Zealand
Website: www.cancernz.org.nz
Tel: 0800 226 237
Provides information and support for people with cancer.

New Zealand Ministry of Health
Website: www.health.govt.nz
Basic advice on diet and exercise – see under the 'Your Health' heading.

INDEX